60 tips

slimming

Marie Borrel

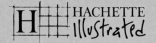

HACHETTE
Illustrated

introduction

the tale of the vanishing weight

The headlines in the press boasting '101 Ways to Lose Your Winter Pounds', piled on over the colder months, herald the arrival of spring more certainly than the first swallow. Many women (and increasingly more men) want to shed those unwanted extra curves. The temptation to go too far too fast is often irresistible. Some people launch themselves onto any old crash diet in the hope that the slimming fairy will witness their dreadful sacrifices and grant them a new slenderness.

Fantasies debunked

Behind the desire to lose weight there often lurks a fantasy. Women often think that losing weight will make all sorts of other things happen. They will have more energy and courage to change their job, they will earn more respect. However, even if the weight sometimes does come off, it is often swiftly regained. This happens for two reasons. First of all, a starved, stressed body compensates for its losses by building up its reserves. When all the problems associated with the weight loss do not magically disappear, we subconsciously prefer to put the pounds and kilos back on rather than confront that harsh reality. Problems must be tackled individually – things just don't go away by themselves.

It is important to remember that losing weight sometimes requires proper medical guidance. There's no problem with losing a few curves before going on holiday: that you can do on your own, as long as you do not have any known health issues. However, if you suffer from any disease (high blood-pressure, diabetes, heart or respiratory problems), it is advisable to ask the advice of a specialist. Likewise, if you have more than ten kilos or one and a half stone to lose, medical guidance is not necessary. However, if you are very overweight you are more likely to have high blood pressure, high blood fats and a high sugar level. A medical examination and blood tests may be sensible.

Questions you should ask yourself

There is nothing wrong with wanting to lose weight in order to feel better about your body and the way you look, to help your body function better and to enjoy the way you move and the clothes you wear. Before you do so, ask yourself a few important questions and answer them honestly. What do you expect from a diet? What is your target weight? Is it just about fashion or is it more to do with how you perceive your body? Although it is good for both mind and body to reach one's ideal weight – the weight at which we feel good aesthetically, emotionally and physically – there is no point in setting an unachievable, wholly elusive target.

The right way to eat

Once you have properly considered and set your objectives, it is time to formulate a plan of attack. Naturally, in order to lose weight you have to eat less. What is most important, however, is to eat better, discover new eating habits and new tastes, reach a compromise between gourmet temptation and contentment with how your body looks. Now's the time to start eating a fresh, healthy and varied diet, enhanced by herbs and spices.

Long-term weight loss does not necessarily involve saying goodbye to the joy of eating. Quite the opposite! It is still part of your daily routine but with modifications. You have to learn how to manage your appetite and your cravings.

Slimming aids: what you can expect

Since the advent of the dietary revolution, a thousand ways to help and support you are out there. On a psychological level, you can start by rethinking the way you feel about yourself, the relationship you have with your image, the reasons why you eat certain things. You might want to try a traditional psychologist or consider other methods, such as hypnosis or NLP (Neuro Linguistic Programming).

On a physical level, exercise is vital. It boosts your energy levels, promotes cell renewal and speeds up elimination of waste. Alternative medicine can also help but don't expect more from it than it is able to provide – no homeopathic remedy or vitamin alone can make you lose weight. The right ones may improve the efficiency of a diet.

Pitfalls to be avoided

It is vital to banish the false belief, often deeply engrained in our minds, that losing weight must involve suffering, as if we need to atone for the original sin of gluttony. Not only can you lose weight without suffering, but in fact, the less you suffer the better the chances of keeping the weight off in the long term. At the same time, it doesn't mean that dieting is all about having fun. It involves a real reappraisal, both psychological and physical, a review of your mindset, lifestyle and eating habits. In order to resist 'cracking' at the first temptation or setback, you need to find a balance that works for you between what your body likes to eat or craves and what is right for it.

It's a real re-education, a serious reprogramming. Realistic slimming is the order of the day, and not the idealized concept portrayed in magazines. It is your diet, your slimness, your method of finding happiness with your body and with others!

how to use this book

This book offers a made-to-measure programme, which will enable you to deal with your own particular problem. It is organized into four sections:

- **A questionnaire** to help you to assess the extent of your problem.
- **The first 20 tips** that will show you how to change your daily life in order to prevent problems and maintain health and fitness.
- **20 slightly more radical tips** that will develop the subject and enable you to cope when problems occur.
- **The final 20 tips** which are intended for more serious cases, when preventative measures and attempted solutions have not worked.

At the end of each section someone with the same problem as you shares his or her experiences.

You can go methodically through the book from tip 1 to 60 putting each piece of advice into practice. Alternatively, you can pick out the recommendations which appear to be best suited to your particular case, or those which fit most easily into your daily routine. Or, finally, you can choose to follow the instructions according to whether you wish to prevent stress problems occuring or cure ones that already exist.

● ● ● FOR YOUR GUIDANCE

> A symbol at the bottom of each page will help you to identify the natural solutions available:

Herbal medicine, aromatherapy, homeopathy, Dr Bach's flower remedies – how natural medicine can help.

Simple exercises – preventing problems by strengthening your body.

Massage and manipulation – how they help to promote well-being.

Healthy eating – all you need to know about the contribution it makes.

Practical tips for your daily life – so that you can prevent instead of having to cure.

Psychology, relaxation, Zen – advice to help you be at peace with yourself and regain serenity.

> A complete programme that will solve all your health problems. Try it!

where do those extra pounds come from?

Read the following statements, think carefully about the problem described, then answer honestly as to whether the statement applies to you or not.

1	I follow strict diets and then give up after a few days.
2	I snack constantly during the day.
3	I skip breakfast.
4	I love fatty and sweet food and don't eat many vegetables or fruit.
5	I don't do any exercise.
6	I can't control my appetite.
7	I have difficulty eliminating toxins – I perspire little and swell in the heat.
8	I have lots of cellulite.
9	I don't like looking in the mirror – I have a complex about my body.
10	I feel guilty when I can't lose any weight
11	I pay lots of attention to fashion.
12	I have a very stressful life.

If you answered YES to at least two of the questions 1 to 4, turn to Tips **1** to **20**.
If you answered YES to at least two of the questions 5 to 8, turn straight to Tips **21** to **40**.
If you answered YES to at least two of the questions 9 to 12, Tips **41** to **60** are the ones to which you must pay most attention.

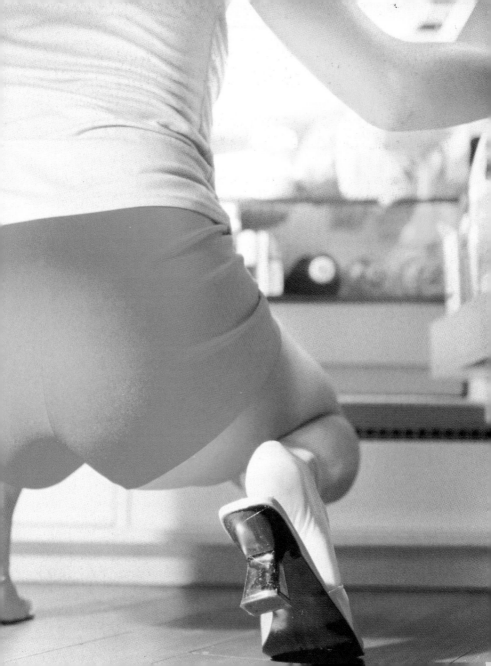

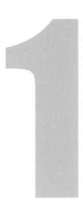

» **Very strict diets are no longer fashionable,** of course, with your scales and notebook to hand to note down every single calorie. The doctors have finally stopped torturing us!

»» But that doesn't mean that you can lose weight by eating whatever you want. **Slimming is still a question of balance** between what you eat and what you expend in energy.

»»» If you want to shed your surplus pounds calmly and without fear of putting them back on, you need to completely re-educate your eating habits. Acquire new habits that can be incorporated into your daily life, not as a punishment, but as a new way of life, **without depriving yourself of the joy of food…**

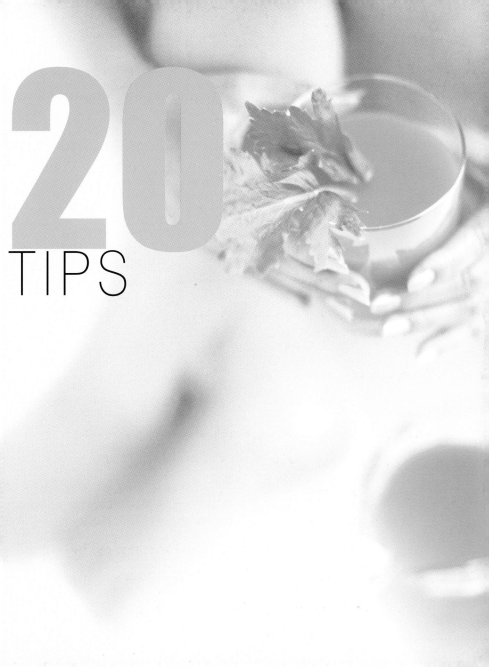

20
TIPS

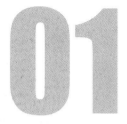

Losing weight, more often than not, involves reducing your food intake. The most important thing is to eat better. Choose different foods, discover new ways of cooking and experiment with new tastes.

eat less, eat better

A surplus balance

If you have already tried very strict diets, you will have noticed one thing: you deprive yourself, you stick at it, you try and try and then... you finally crack and give up. Of course, the pounds and kilos drop off, as if a reward for your stoicism, but then they make a swift return, as if a punishment for your fickleness.

In general, we accumulate an impressive number of lost pounds and kilos over

● ● ● DID YOU KNOW?

> Your body is a valuable and permanent companion, an incredibly complex machine. It may suffer the odd hiccup, but you should look upon it as a friend who supports you through the hard times.

> You will find it easier to enjoy feeding your body with what is good for it and avoiding the things that are bad for it.

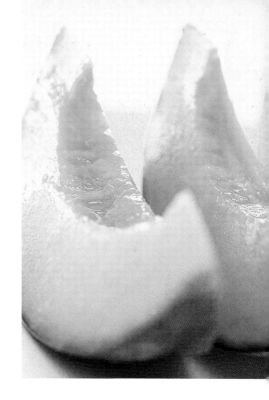

the years but an even a more impressive number of them are regained. The balance of payments is zero at best but more likely a surplus.

A few tricks that really work…

Wipe the slate clean and make a fresh start! First of all, focus your attention on what you can have rather than what you can't have. Instead of saying: 'I mustn't eat jam', say to yourself, 'I can enjoy all the fresh summer fruits from the market.' Similarly, instead of giving up entirely on fried food, try treating yourself to the new vegetable oils in the supermarkets. This will open up your horizons to new, even unexpected, pleasures.

Everything revolves around one simple rule: nothing is forbidden, apart from sweets (see Tip 5) and cooked fats (see Tip 6). And try to give priority to foods that are high in nutrition and low in calories: especially vegetables, then fruits, fish, low-fat dairy products etc.

KEY FACTS

If you want to lose weight in the long term, change your eating habits.

Focus on those foods that are good for you and you will discover new pleasures.

Focus attention on nutritious, low-calorie foods.

Our bodies are equipped with a highly refined guidance system: the appetite. Hunger, dietary whims and cravings are normally a function of our needs. Learn to reconnect with your infallible guide.

02

listen to your appetite

It's your brain that's hungry

For decades, hunger was explained as an empty space in the stomach. Then it was thought to be a drop in blood-sugar levels. Today we know that it is our brain that feels hunger and monitors the level of our energy reserves. When these reserves get low, the brain triggers the release of the signs of hunger (salivation, gnawing feeling in the stomach, etc.) to prompt us to eat.

● ● ● DID YOU KNOW?

> If all foods tasted the same we would find it difficult to vary our diet. Our taste buds are highly sophisticated, with thousands of specific receptors which are relayed by our sense of smell and vision.

> An aromatic, attractively presented dish goes down better with our taste buds than dreary or bland food.

Time to rethink

Since our body has a constant need for energy, our brain, the organ in control of our impulses and emotions, supplies it continuously. No surprise, then, that the hunger process is sometimes disrupted by strong emotions urging us to eat when our body does not need it, or, conversely, urging us to stop eating and starve ourselves.

If you want to separate the 'correct' information from the 'disrupted' messages, you need to re-educate your appetite. For example, make yourself wait for a while between the time when the desire to eat strikes and the time when you actually put food in your mouth. Ten minutes is enough to start with: relax, concentrate on what is happening in your body and listen to your emotions. This is often enough time for purely emotional cravings to subside.

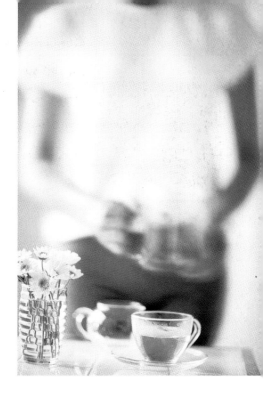

> Our personal tastes are influenced by our taste memory: the more varied our diet, the richer our tastes. This is the case from our earliest years. It's time to widen your taste horizons.

KEY FACTS

✳ It is our brain that controls our appetite and triggers our hunger pangs.

✳ It's the brain that controls our emotions, so it's hardly surprising that it influences our appetite.

✳ Re-educate your appetite in order to be able to trust it.

03

avoid faddy diets

Diets flourish in the spring, popping up like daisies in fields – the dissociated diet, the Atkins diet, the Beverly Hills diet. The media sing their praises before highlighting their more negative sides. It's generally advisable to avoid them in the first place.

Malnourished, pale and tired

A few decades ago, magazines sang the praises of the dissociated diet, which advocated eating fruit one day, vegetables the next and meat the next. You could lose weight quickly due to the difficulty of eating any really large quantity of the same food in one day. However, dieters swiftly became malnourished, pale and tired. Once they stopped dieting, they quickly put the weight back on. The same scenario was repeated over the years with the Mayot diet (loads of eggs, few vegetables, no carbohydrates or fats at all) and the Beverly Hills diet (fruit only).

● ● ● DID YOU KNOW?

> Meal substitutes are powders or soups designed to replace a full meal. They are enriched with nutrients to avoid serious malnourishment. However, their use should be restricted. A meal substituted is really only better than a meal skipped or inappropriate snacking.

> Don't just eat substitutes – they won't give you the proper nutritional benefits and may disturb your dietary pattern. The general advice is to limit your intake of them to one per day, two at the most.

The popular Atkins diet allows you to eat protein (eggs, meat, fish) and fats without restriction but forbids carbohydrates, fruit and vegetables as well as sugar. No sugar in the diet means no insulin is released and the body starts to break down fat. This leads to the formation of 'ketone bodies' which tend to reduce appetite. The protein and fat help you to feel full. Although dieticians point out that the diet is deficient in fibre and micro-nutrients and may raise blood cholesterol, many dieters have found it effective and will put up with the constipation.

Slowly but surely...

These diets go out of fashion very quickly, not only because they are generally ineffective, but also because they are responsible for the well known yo-yo effect, together with nutritional deficiencies, cellular stress and other side effects. If you want to lose weight and keep it off, get used to the idea that speed is not compatible with durability. It's better to lose a few pounds or a kilo a week, whilst adhering to good eating habits, than to lose large amounts in a few days, only to put it all – and more – back on again. Early rapid weight loss is due to loss of glycogen (stored sugar) in the kidneys and protein breakdown with accompanying water loss. After 3-4 weeks weight loss slows.

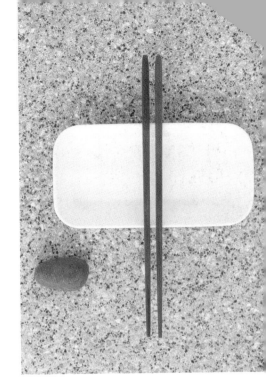

KEY FACTS

* Faddy diets are best avoided.

* If you lose the pounds or kilos quickly, you'll put them back on even more swiftly.

* When it comes to slimming, durability is not compatible with speed. Lose small amounts of weight steadily.

04

drink plenty of water

In order to lose weight, you also need to help your body eliminate waste. Add to this the fact that the process by which your body loses fat causes the production of extra toxins. So drinking enough water is vital.

A surplus of waste

Our body is composed of 70% water. All our cells bathe in an interstitial liquid through which pass both the nutrients they need and the waste they produce. Water is also the main component of our body liquids: blood, lymph, etc. Even our bones, so dry and solid in appearance, have a water content of around 30%. If it is vital for everybody to drink water, it's even more important when

● ● ● DID YOU KNOW?

> The minerals contained in mineral water generally have high bioavailability. This means that the body can absorb and use them easily. The same is not true of all foods.

> In order to lose weight, choose a water that is low in sodium and rich in magnesium and sulphates. Take a good look at the label, which states the precise mineral composition.

you are on a weight-reducing diet, when the body is forced to draw on its fat deposits to find the energy it needs. To do this it has to perform metabolic processes that in turn produce toxins. So you must drink plenty of water to help the emunctory organs (principally the kidneys and liver) to flush out these surplus toxins.

Calorie-free minerals

Furthermore, while we are slimming, we need to nourish our body differently: we may be reducing our energy intake, but we should maintain, even increase our nutritional intake (vitamins, minerals, etc.). Water is rich in minerals and trace elements, all for zero calories. Make the most of it. Some mineral waters are reputed to aid slimming. Let's be clear about this – none of them can actually make you lose weight! Some fruit juices and carbonated drinks can be high in calories. Drinking flavoured or sparkling water gives fluid and taste without the extra calories.

As a general rule, the recommended intake of water is one and a half litres or two and a half pints of water per day.

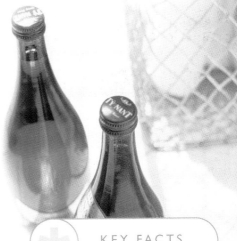

> Don't always drink the same water, particularly if it is highly mineralized (no more than one month). Vary the brands to vary your mineral intake.

KEY FACTS

⬧ Drink plenty of water when you are on a diet.

⬧ The reduction of fat generates waste products that the body needs to flush out.

⬧ Mineral waters contain the nutritional benefits without the calories.

05

You've stopped taking white sugar in your coffee and you no longer add it to your cereal. But did you know that many other foods contain sugar? An ordinary glass of a fizzy drink contains the equivalent of 5 to 6 spoonfuls!

avoid those hidden sugars

Cakes, sweets, sauces and soups etc.

Refined white sugar is the only food that we can cut out of our diets without risking deficiencies. Even better, it is recommended that everyone give it up, since it is the source of many problems. It is extracted from sugar beet or sugar cane by a refining process that destroys all the nutrients it contains. Sugar needs certain micronutrients to be assimilated, metabolised or used by the body.

● ● ● DID YOU KNOW?

> Sugar is the first taste to incite pleasure in a newborn baby. It is a source of reassurance and consolation. If you feel you need it, try synthetic sweeteners, which do not contain any nutrients (apart from the amino acids of which they are formed) and are very low in calories.

> As part of a diet, artificial sweeteners allow us to satisfy our cravings for sugar without tipping the scales.

Refined sugar is often hidden in industrially manufactured products, such as fizzy drinks, cakes, sweets and sauces.

Deficiencies as well as pounds!

If you don't watch out you can end up absorbing well over the 25g (1 oz) of fast sugar our bodies need every day without even realizing it. It is this excess of sugar that is immediately stored by the body as fat and is easily and quickly absorbed.

Also, refined sugar needs certain micronutrients to be assimilated, specifically B group vitamins and chromium. Any nutrients it may itself have contained are destroyed in the refining process. So the body has to draw on its own reserves to find these substances. Which means you risk nutritional deficiencies as well as weight gain!

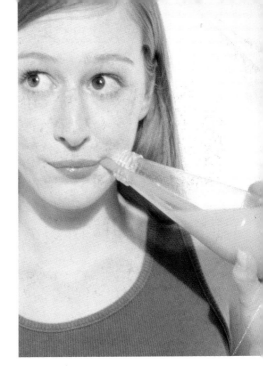

> But be careful – it's better to try to change the way you relate to sugar, for example by learning to appreciate unsweetened coffee and herbal teas, rather than taking systematic recourse to sweeteners.

KEY FACTS

* White sugar is the only food that we should cut from our diet.

* The body must draw on its own nutritional reserves to metabolise it, which means a risk of deficiencies.

* Watch out for hidden sugar in fizzy drinks, cakes, sweets and sauces.

06

choose 'good' fats

Weight-reducing diets have long dictated that we reduce our fat intake to a minimum, and even cut it out completely. But fat is vital for our bodies to function. It's important to find the right balance and not eat just any fat.

Brain suppleness

In so far as calories are concerned, all fats are the same. In their natural state, in plants and living beings, fats constitute a sort of reservoir where maximum energy is stored in minimum space. Fatty substances also have the highest calorie content: 9 calories per gram compared to 3 or 4 per gram of carbohydrate. They should not therefore be excluded from your diet, because doing so would be risking serious deficiencies. The membranes of our cells are composed mainly by fats in order to maintain elasticity, so that information can pass through them easily. If we do not eat enough fatty substances, the cell walls become rigid and information does not pass smoothly from one cell to the other. Little by little, the entire body slows down and begins to age prematurely, particularly the brain and the nervous system.

Two tablespoons a day

If you want to lose weight, you should limit your fat intake and give priority to vegetable oils. These contain the essential fatty acids (mono and polyunsaturates) that nourish the cell walls. Eat them uncooked wherever possible, since certain fatty acids are fragile and are destroyed by heat. But, steer well clear of animal fats (butter, fatty cheeses, fatty meats) that contain saturated fatty acids

which are bad for your arteries. Only fish contains good fatty acids. As part of a strict diet, you can eat a tablespoonful of uncooked oil per meal. Vary the sources. You will benefit from the different flavours and compositions of the essential fatty acids of olive, grapeseed, sunflower, corn and sesame oils.

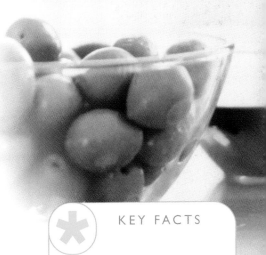

> Animal fats contain saturated fatty acids. These can do damage to your arteries. Buy a variety of vegetable oils to add flavour and interest to your food.

No more boring diets based on boiled vegetables! You really can get cooking: combine, and enjoy balancing, different tastes and a real bouquet of flavours, which can still be healthy.

07

opt for healthy cooking methods

The champion of all cooking categories: braising

This is an ideal way of cooking: all the flavour, vitamins and minerals are retained and no fat is needed. Also, because the temperature remains below 100°C (200°F) it doesn't destroy the food and, as you eat the cooking juices along with the rest of the dish, no nutrients are lost. This method is suitable for

DID YOU KNOW?

> Take care with grills and barbecues. These methods do not require any additional fat and, even better, fats hidden in the meat dissolve. But these high cooking temperatures generate new, highly toxic molecules.

> Don't eat large quantities of grilled meat and above all, don't eat the charred bits. Avoid foods touching the flame during cooking.

lean meats, poultry, vegetables and fruits. Herbs and spices are welcome additions. Ideally, choose a stainless steel or a cast-iron casserole dish and only lightly peel organic vegetables to retain the maximum nutrients. Fish is best cooked in a foil parcel in a warm oven. If you add acid ingredients (lemon, tomatoes, etc.) use greaseproof paper rather than foil to avoid any seepage of the metallic micro-particles into the food.

Boil or steam

Boiling is more efficient in slimming terms, but not in so far as concerns nutrition, because vitamins and minerals are left in the cooking water. If you want to get the last drop out of what you eat, don't throw this water away: use it to make soups or as the base of light sauces. On the other hand, if you are cooking vegetables that might have been treated with chemicals, throw the water away. You might lose the vitamins this way, but at least you won't congest your body with pollutants (nitrates, pesticides, etc.). Steaming better conserves the nutritional content of food as long as the cooking temperature does not exceed 100°C (200°F).

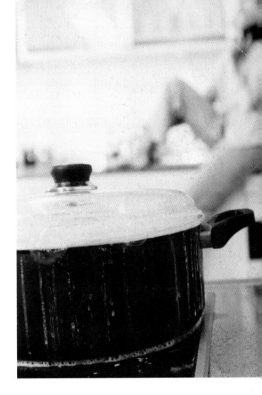

KEY FACTS

* Learn to cook in a healthy, flavoursome, low-calorie way.

* The best cooking methods are braising and steaming in foil over a low flame.

* Take care with grills and barbeques: combustion creates toxic molecules.

Even when you are on a diet, your body needs all the nutrients for it to continue functioning properly. Don't deprive it of the elements it needs, just get rid of what it doesn't need...

08

eat a balanced diet

Play 4-2-1

Going on a diet? There's no better time to learn the basics of a balanced diet. When you eat too much your body always, or nearly always, ends up getting what it needs from your food intake, although it may also find it harder to rid itself of the surpluses and substances it doesn't need. But when you are reducing your food intake, there is a risk that it

● ● ● DID YOU KNOW?

> Carbohydrates are also high in fibre. They are vital on several counts.
● First of all, they increase the volume of stools and facilitate digestion. Diets too high in protein and deficient in fruit, cereals and vegetables result in stubborn constipation.

● Secondly, carbohydrates make you feel fuller.

will run short on some elements. So it's important to make sure that your diet is well balanced.

It can be difficult to strike the right balance. We all need proteins (meats, eggs, fish, etc.), carbohydrates (cereals, leguminous plants, potatoes, vegetables, fruits), and fats (oils, butter, hidden fats). Every day, make sure your diet provides four parts carbohydrate for every two parts proteins and one part fat. That's the 4-2-1 rule.

Basic advice

First of all, don't cut out any one food category completely (with the exception of white sugar). Aside from any nutritional deficiencies, this type of sacrifice leads to frustration… and so to transgression.

Next, don't reduce the overall volume too drastically. Aim to choose foods that have both the bulk and the nutrition, for fewer calories (tomatoes, green salad, raw vegetables, etc.).

Finally, try to eat these types of food in combination with a richer food (potatoes, meat, cheese).

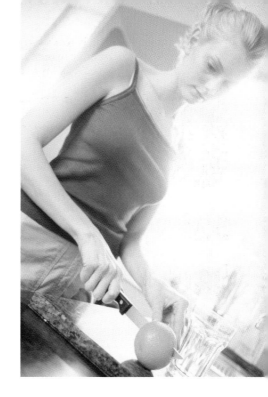

KEY FACTS

* A weight-reducing diet is an ideal opportunity to discover a new dietary balance.

* You need to eat 4 portions of carbohydrates for every 2 of protein and 1 of fat.

* Don't cut out any one category of food completely.

09

add
vitamins

Other obligatory guests at our daily meal are micronutrients: vitamins, minerals and trace elements. Without them, we risk being overcome by tiredness and cracking at the first opportunity. A healthy diet is a vitamin rich diet.

Minute but vital

Our bodies have no way of manufacturing these micronutrients. Although present in infinitesimal quantities, they are vital for the millions of metabolic reactions our bodies need to perform every minute to maintain life. We get vitamins, minerals and trace elements from the food we eat. If your intake is too low, biochemical reactions can fail to function properly, you body flags and tiredness sets in. In the long term, more serious problems may arise.

Fresh and varied

The most important thing, to be sure of giving your body all the micronutrients it needs despite dietary restrictions, is to vary your diet. Eat as many untreated fresh products as you can (fruits, vegetables, fish and poultry). Don't keep your fruits and vegetables too long because some vitamins oxidize on exposure to air and light. A potato, for example, loses up to 90% of its vitamin C in this way. If you drink fresh fruit juices, consume them immediately. If you buy organic or untreated fruits and vegetables, peel them as little as possible – most of the vitamins are concentrated in the skin, except, of course, in the case of citrus fruits, such as oranges and grapefruit.

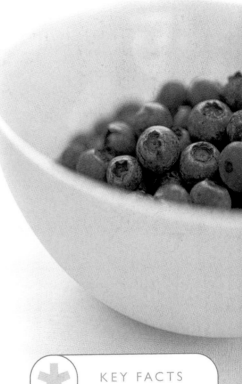

> What's more, pollutants (insecticides, pesticides, etc.) have a tendancy to collect in milk fat, so skimmed milk and low-fat dairy products can also be more healthy.

KEY FACTS

* Take care not to miss out on vitamins, minerals and trace elements.

* Choose fresh, untreated products and don't keep foods for too long.

* Avoid diet foods, apart from low-fat dairy products.

10 forget about calories

For many years slimming diets were synonymous with calorie counting. Nowadays, nutritionists know that a calorie of sausage is not the same as a calorie of apple...

Between 600 and 1,500 calories a day: a calorie is a unit that measures the energy content of a food. Calories are calculated by measuring the time it takes to burn a specific quantity of matter under predetermined atmospheric conditions. This unit of measurement, however, does not give any idea of the composition of the food.

Each food is assimilated at its own rate: we know that the body does not use 100g (4oz) of oil in the same way as 100g (4oz) of cabbage, 100g (4oz) of fish, 100g (4oz) of apple, 100g (4oz) of sugar or 100g (4oz) of egg white. Some nutrients are easily stored while others require an effort on the part of the body. Some are assimilated easily while other need metabolic operations that themselves, in turn, consume energy. The result is not always the same when they reach the finishing line!

● ● ● DID YOU KNOW?

> The average calorie intake of a 65 kg adult is between 2,000 and 2,500 calories per day. When you are on a diet, this intake should be 600 to 1,500 calories. But these must still be distributed in a balanced way. Do note that the lower the intake, the harder it is to maintain a balanced diet.

KEY FACTS

* The calorie is a unit for measuring the energy content of a food.

* All calories are not the same.

* It's better to focus on a balanced diet.

11 plan for your hunger pangs

A sudden pang of hunger, a craving for a snack? Make sure you don't crack and end up eating just anything. Prepare yourself some low-fat snacks and keep them to hand for when you need them.

Sudden, overpowering, overwhelming hunger: this is our greatest fear when dieting… that craving for a snack that suddenly grips you. You make a dash for the fridge and eat whatever you find which, more often than not, is something you shouldn't be eating: a cake, a piece of cheese, some chocolate. Avoid giving in to the temptation to snack on foods that will upset the balance and make you feel guilty by planning ahead.

Courgettes, prawns and white cheese: try preparing some little snacks that you can keep to hand 'just in case'. Hard-boiled eggs, boiled prawns, celery or carrot sticks, a bowl of low-fat cheese with lemon and basil, for example. Also good as a snack are grilled vegetables (tomatoes, courgettes, peppers, etc.) conserved in a spoonful of oil.

KEY FACTS

* It's a good idea to have some snacks ready to hand.

* Hard boil some eggs, chop up some vegetable sticks.

* Always serve your snack on a plate so that you can keep track of what you eat.

12 have a good breakfast

It's the first meal of the day, so don't skip it just because you are on a diet. That doesn't mean that then you can eat what you like... a little discipline is required.

Recharge your batteries

During the night, our body valiantly carries on performing its tasks. Some functions shut down while others are at their peak of activity, so, when we wake up in the morning we are running on empty. We need a battery recharge and a full tank to get going in the morning or run the risk of running out of energy during the morning, then cracking and eating whatever is at hand.

A low-fat breakfast

A good breakfast should provide the body with all the nutrients – fats, carbohydrates, proteins, vitamins, minerals and trace elements. But, not in just any old form. Avoid fast sugars (jam, honey, white sugar, corn flakes). Watch out for hidden fats (pastries, croissants).

Make the right choices

For example: two slices of brown bread, a little butter (a teaspoonful), a slice of cooked ham or a boiled egg, a piece of fruit or a glass fresh fruit juice, a low-fat yoghurt or some skimmed milk with tea or a herbal infusion. For a reasonable amount of calories, your body will have what it needs to start the day without tiredness or deficiency, and will wait patiently for lunchtime.

KEY FACTS

* Breakfast is a vital meal for recharging your body's batteries after its night's work.

* It should represent one quarter of your daily food intake.

* It should provide you with all the nutrients (proteins, carbohydrates, fats, vitamins, minerals and trace elements), as well as water.

> This is why infusions constitute a good breakfast drink. You can have several cups without worrying about your nerves or addiction, as you would with coffee.

13

don't skip meals

Skipping a meal to compensate for the previous day's overindulgence is a really bad idea if you want to lose weight in the long term. You must eat regularly.

Body stress

Don't skip meals, as you are more likely to feel hungry and be tempted to fill up on high-calorie snacks. Starving the body can of course be set off against any excess from the previous meal. But this offset is illusory. Firstly, when deprived of all nourishment, the body suffers stress and will simply build up a reserve the next time you eat, in case it happens again. So you may gain a little extra weight rather than actually losing any.

Metabolic slowdown

These nutritional imbalances, if repeated too often, encourage your body to get into the habit of functioning to a minimum. Your body reduces its outgoings to avoid risking a deficiency, and in this way, you gradually slow down your metabolism. Some people reduce their food intake over a period of years until they are living on a calorie intake that is the other side of restrictive. If you feel the need to take a break after an over-indulgent or over-alcoholic evening, stick to eating lightly for the next meal: a vegetable soup, a green salad, a piece of fruit. Cut back... but don't cut out!

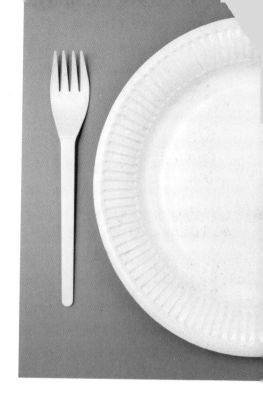

> Furthermore, the body, stressed by these privations, quickly replaces the lost pounds or kilos and increases its tendency to build up permanent reserves.

KEY FACTS

* Skipping meals just simply doesn't work.

* Think before you eat.

* It's better to eat very lightly, for example, soup, salad or a piece of fruit.

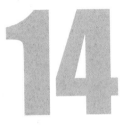

Eating a balanced diet is vital to lose weight. But it is even more efficient to balance your meals by organizing them around low-fat foods: these provide plenty of nutrients and few calories.

14

choose
lighter foods

Foods you can eat in any quantity

Vegetables, fruits and low-fat dairy products contain little fat and hidden sugar. They are full of water and stuffed with micronutrients. You can eat them in great quantities without any risk and they quickly make you feel full. Some of them speed up diuresis and help to flush out water accumulated in the tissues. Others help to ease congestion in the liver, maintain the nervous system and improve digestion. The result? A diet that will make you lose weight while helping your body to carry out its daily tasks.

You choose

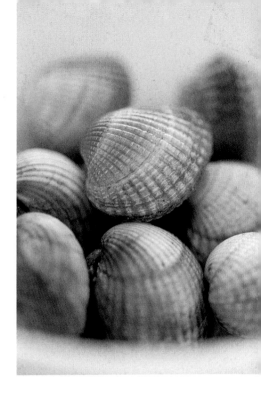

Vegetables: tomatoes, cucumbers, courgettes/zucchini, peppers, green salad, artichokes, aubergines/egg plant and mushrooms.

Fruits: citrus fruits (oranges, grapefruit etc), strawberries, peaches (rich in vitamin C).

Dairy products: low-fat yoghurts (with no added sugar or with sweetener), low-fat white cheese.

Meats: poultry, fillet steak, pork fillet, veal (escalope or extra-lean joint).

Fish and seafood: sole, sea bass, coley, whiting, shellfish and seafood.

> Also, eat vegetables, fruit and dairy products in reasonable quantities. You should not feel too full when you leave the table.

KEY FACTS

* Some foods are very low in calories and yet still very high in nutrients.

* These foods help the body to function while at the same time aiding weight loss.

* Organize your meals around a high-protein food.

15 allow yourself a few treats

You don't have to live like a monk to lose weight! The pleasure of the palate is an essential part of your diet. Taking pleasure in eating makes your metabolism more efficient and speeds up your digestion.

Light, healthy – and good for you! The same foods can have a different impact on your body according to whether they are combined in a way that is pleasant or unpleasant. The pleasure you experience when you eat can increase your base metabolism. Not enough, of course, to compensate for all our indulgences, but to a limited extent. It is better to eat in a way that is light, healthy and enjoyable, than light, healthy and tasteless.

The metabolic role of pleasure: according to research carried out by Stylianos Nicolaïdis at the French National Centre for Scientific Research, not only do the smell, colour and taste of food tell us that a food is edible, they also have an impact on our digestive system and hormones. Identical foods can have a different impact on the body according to how much we want to eat them... more, or less, pleasure!

KEY FACTS

* The pleasure of eating plays a vital role in our metabolism.

✳ Eat light and healthy foods that you really enjoy as much as possible.

16 don't turn down invitations

Going on a diet shouldn't be like taking holy orders. Conviviality is an essential part of the pleasure of eating, of sharing. Follow these simple rules to prevent invitations becoming mental torture.

Avoid compulsive compensations: there is nothing sadder than denying yourself a night out on the pretext that you are on a diet. You can't get used to a new attitude to eating unless you carry on living normally. This is vital if you don't want the briefest outing to become synonymous with compulsive compensation and regained pounds.

A few tricks that really work: avoid the cocktail snacks, don't eat too much bread and don't have a second helping. Watch how much alcohol you drink, avoid sugary aperitifs and don't have more than one or sometimes two glasses of wine. In restaurants, choose a vegetable-based starter and a fish main course. Skip dessert and watch how much you drink. When entertaining, prepare a light menu and take particular care over flavours and presentation.

● ● ● DID YOU KNOW?

> Buffets are particularly treacherous, because it's difficult to keep track of what you are eating when you are eating little bits and pieces. Try to get a plate and serve yourself so that you can gauge exactly how much you are eating. Keep an eye on your sugar and alcohol intake.

KEY FACTS

* When you are changing the way you relate to food you must continue to lead a normal life.

* Watch your sugar and alcohol intake.

* Choose vegetables, lean meat and fish.

17

consider protein supplements

Protein supplement products can be bought over the counter at any pharmacy. Using them is not entirely free of danger or disadvantages. They should be used only under medical supervision .

Only for severe obesity

Of course hyper-protein products in sachet form make you lose weight quickly, but you must be careful because they are not without their dangers. Although the weight loss is rapid, final weight loss does not exceed that of a longer-term, balanced diet. Also, the side-effects can be severe: cardio-vascular, kidney, psychiatric problems; digestion,

●●● DID YOU KNOW? ─────

> Eating a lot of protein enables weight loss without losing muscle mass. Also, these foods require the body to work quite hard to metabolize them.

> Proteins consume up to 25% of their calorific value. So, an almost total absence of carbohydrate forces the body to draw on its fat reserves.

behavioural issues; hypoglycaemia, low blood pressure and irregular periods. Above all, this treatment is only suitable for severe obesity, administered in a hospital environment.

4 or 5 days maximum

If, however, you want to jump-start your weight-loss regime, you can increase your animal protein intake and cut out all carbohydrates (i.e. bread, pasta, rice, sugar). But be careful – don't do it for more than 4 or 5 days. Eat only lean meats, fish, seafood and shellfish, and some low-calorie, low-carbohydrate vegetables (i.e. cucumbers, green salad, tomatoes), reducing your fat intake to an absolute minimum. After 4 or 5 days, reintroduce the other foods in these successive stages: other vegetables, fruits, low-fat dairy products and finally the slow carbohydrates.

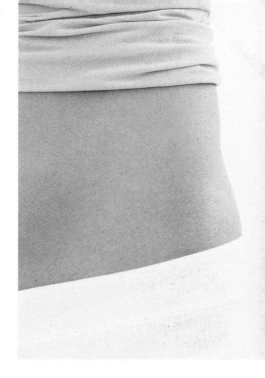

> The body also provides the organs, and particularly the brain, with the sugar it needs, leading to immediate weight loss.

KEY FACTS

* Protein treatment sachets require medical supervision.

* When you start your diet you can increase the quantity of proteins and exclude (or almost exclude) carbohydrates.

* Be careful! Don't exceed 4 or 5 days of this treatment.

Naturopaths recommend a natural detox diet at the start of every new season to help the body rid itself of waste. You might also lose a few pounds or kilos on the way.

18

the twice-yearly mono-diet

Tune into the seasons

An accumulation of toxins in the tissue makes cellulite worse. So thorough elimination is vital for successful slimming. It is also good for helping the body to maintain the action of the excretory organs (liver, kidneys, lungs, skin, intestines).

Make the process more pleasant by following the advice of the naturopaths who recommend a two- to three-day mono-diet around the time of the changes of the seasons. This is particularly advisable at the time of the equinoxes (from winter to spring and summer to autumn).

Strawberries in summer, grapes in the autumn

In the spring, go on a mono-diet of strawberries: for two days, three at the most, just eat strawberries. You can eat as much of them as you want, as long as you don't add any unwanted calories (sugar, cream etc.). Strawberries are low in sugar but very high in vitamins (particularly vitamin C). They have a purifying effect on the liver.

At the start of the autumn, go on a grape mono-diet: follow the same procedure, but replacing the strawberries with grapes. More sugary and higher in calories, grapes are a natural diuretic and a mild laxative. They also contain antioxidants.

dairy products and slow carbohydrates and eat just fruit and vegetables on the day before you start the diet. After the diet, start to reintroduce foods gradually, in the reverse order.

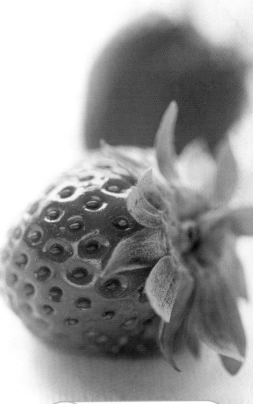

KEY FACTS

A mono-diet will help your body to eliminate toxins.

Strawberries in the spring and grapes in the autumn.

* Exceed 3 days and run the risk of counter-productive deficiencies.

19

eat at the right time

Our body has an internal clock and our metabolism is regulated by regular cycles. According to advocates of chrononutrition, if we learn to respect these cycles slimming will be easier.

Chronobiology and chrononutrition

According to chronobiology, the effect a food has on our body varies according to the time of day when we eat it. Chronobiology is a branch of science that studies biological rhythms. For example, our body uses fats to manufacture the cell walls in the morning, so chronobiologists maintain it needs sugars to compensate for the energy loss of the day in the middle of the afternoon. It is towards midday that it builds up its store of protein reserves. Chrono-nutrition was the result of these discoveries. It centres around trying to give the body what it needs, at the time when it needs it, to help it to get rid of superfluous waste.

A typical day

In the words of Dr Delabos, a specialist in chrononutrition: 'In order to lose weight, you need to eat fats in the morning, have a big meal at lunchtime, a light snack in the afternoon and eat as lightly as possible in the evening.' He advises the following:

• **breakfast:** carbohydrates and fats (bread, butter, cheese, white cheese, egg and bacon) with tea or an infusion. But no fast sugars (white sugar, jam, honey).

• **lunch:** proteins and carbohydrates. The ideal is a single course (meat and pasta, fish and potatoes, pork and lentils) with no starter, cheese or dessert.

• **snack:** faster sugars and vegetable fats (olives, dried fruits), but no bread and butter or pastries, of course.

• **dinner:** a meal of fruits, or a little fish and green vegetables, limiting quantities to an absolute minimum.

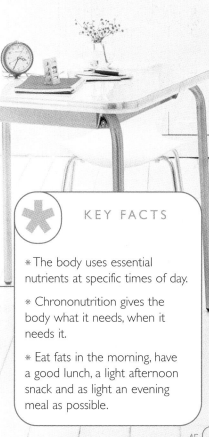

> Conversely, a barrel-shaped figure, (slim arms and legs with a chubby tummy) is a sign of too much starchy food. This is why an accurate assessment of your figure, with a series of measurements, is more important in their eyes than your weight alone.

KEY FACTS

* The body uses essential nutrients at specific times of day.

* Chrononutrition gives the body what it needs, when it needs it.

* Eat fats in the morning, have a good lunch, a light afternoon snack and as light an evening meal as possible.

20 know how to shop

When you're on a diet, your regime starts in the supermarket. The surest way of not breaking your diet when you're at home is to buy just what you need and nothing extra, but still to do it with pleasure.

Eat before you shop: don't go shopping when you're starving hungry. Filling your trolley with everything in reach is more likely to happen on an empty stomach. Buy fresh produce from your local fruit and vegetable shop as often as you can. There you won't be tempted by factory-prepared foods packed with sugar and hidden fats.

Avoid that empty cupboard feeling: force yourself not to buy anything that might make you break your diet, but don't end up with bare cupboards as dull as a circus without a clown! Concentrate on ingredients that you like and that you can incorporate into your meals. Above all, don't fall into the empty cupboard trap. That will just mean you are forced to do a quick shop, buying whatever you can, wherever you can.

KEY FACTS

* Never go shopping on an empty stomach.

* Use a local fruit and vegetable shop rather than a supermarket.

* Buy ingredients you like and that you are allowed to eat.

case study

'I started to put on weight when I was eight years old. I went through a bit of a bulimic phase, brought on by the tense atmosphere at home. I had a really sweet tooth and loved sugary dishes and rich food that made me feel full. The pounds I accumulated over the course of a decade were really difficult to shed later. I did what everybody did: the first diet worked like a charm, and then there was the rapid weight regain, followed by despair and starting again…until the day I found a dietician who spoke to me differently. She refused to tell me everything I couldn't eat, but she did take delight in telling me everything I could eat. I learned to enjoy going to the market in the morning, returning with fresh fruit and vegetables, freshly caught fish… I set about cooking, me, who used to only like slapping pasta on a plate. I started to develop a finer palate, enjoy more varied tastes. I lost weight little by little: it was like a 'lucky side-effect' of my new way of eating.'

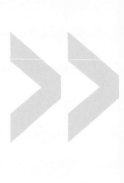

21

» **There's no miracle product, drug or technique** that can make you lose weight without making an effort and without changing your behaviour. But that doesn't mean that nothing can help you and support you in your venture.

»» **Plants, homeopathy, Chinese medicine, sport, algae, massage**… are all allies that you can get on your side.

»»» When it comes to beauty, **nature has thought of everything, even our whims.** Trust nature and it will help you without any risk, which is more than can be said for drugs (chemical appetite suppressants, diuretics) some of which have been withdrawn from the market as they are potentially dangerous.

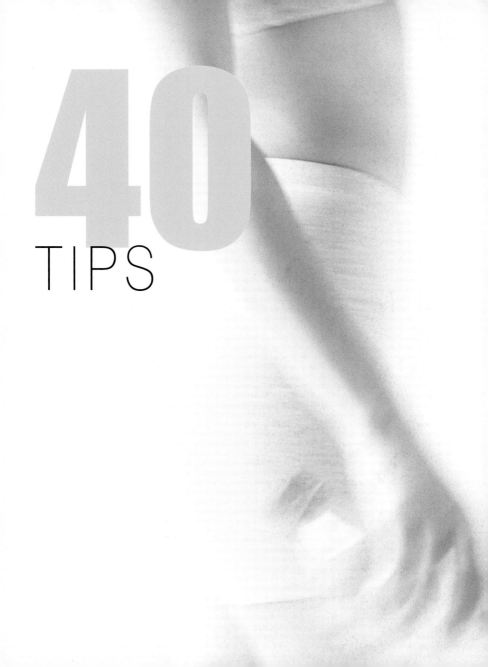

40
TIPS

21

use plants to get rid of cellulite

Plants – the biggest sellers at the pharmacy.
They have draining and diuretic qualities,
and can moderate the appetite.
Some plants can even stimulate the action
of the hormones and help to clear
accumulated cellulite.

Orange-peel skin and water retention

Plants are held to be particularly efficient when the weight gain is the result of water retention or cellulite. Real cellulite is an inflammation of the subcutaneous tissues caused by an accumulation of toxins, fats and water. Some medicinal plants increase the volume of urine, while others can decongest the tissue. As part of a slimming programme,

●●● DID YOU KNOW?

> There are plant-based anti-cellulite creams available on the market: ivy, algae, horse chestnut etc. They work on the blood and lymphatic circulation. They often contain caffeine, which helps to break down localized areas of cellulite.

> These creams can't perform miracles but they can provide help in the battle many women wage against cellulite. Use them as part of your beauty programme.

they are best taken in the form of herbal teas. This is a good way of increasing the amount of liquid you drink almost without noticing it. Don't add sugar. If you don't like the taste, add herbs with a sweeter taste to your infusion (such as verbena, citronella or lemon balm).

Plants that 'work'

• **Pilosella:** this is a very effective diuretic. It helps to eliminate urea. Add around 50 g (2 oz) to a litre (1³/₄ pints) of boiling water, leave to stand for a quarter of an hour. Drink 3 cups per day.
• **Fennel root:** this contains potassium and flavonoids, which are the properties that reduce congestion. Add around 25 g (1 oz) to a litre (1³/₄ pints) of cold water. Boil for 5 minutes and then leave to stand for 10 minutes. Drink 1 cup before every meal.
• **Orthosiphon:** this is a very powerful diuretic that helps the elimination of

many types of waste (urea, uric acid, excess acidity). Add one tablespoonful to 250 ml (8 fl oz) of boiling water. Leave to stand for 10 minutes. Drink 3 cups per day.

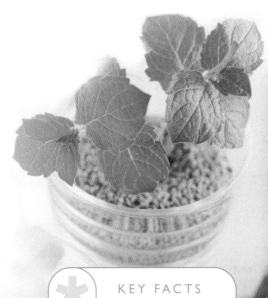

> The action of anti-cellulite creams is improved by massage, which you should do for 5 minutes before and after application.

KEY FACTS

* Plants help to ease congestion in the tissue and reduce areas of cellulite.

* Try pilosella, fennel root and orthosiphon.

* Plant-based creams need to be applied over a sufficiently long period.

These marine plants have the ability to simulate the function of hormones, and particularly of the thyroid gland. People who tend to put on weight often suffer from an under-active thyroid gland.

22

discover the benefits of algae

Vegetable palm and the war on weight

Algae are a highly prized ingredient in the cosmetics industry. These marine plants continuously filter the liquid in which they live to obtain nourishment. In the process, they retain numerous substances that are vital to keep us healthy and slim – iodine, of course, but also vitamins, minerals, amino acids and trace elements. They are an incomparably rich source. Among the 25,000 recorded varieties are the brown algae which provide the vegetable palm used in the weight-loss war.

Marine iodine and the thyroid gland

It is above all their richness in iodine that gives some algae their slimming properties, particularly fucus and laminaria. Iodine is the most important fuel source of the thyroid gland. When the thyroid gland is working slowly, the metabolism gets lazy and the body runs on minimum output, storing as much as it can. Fucus and laminaria supply the body with a surplus of marine iodine that can help to boost the thyroid gland and increase expenditure. Also, these algae stimulate blood and lymphatic circulation, thereby helping to eliminate toxins and decongest areas affected by cellulite.

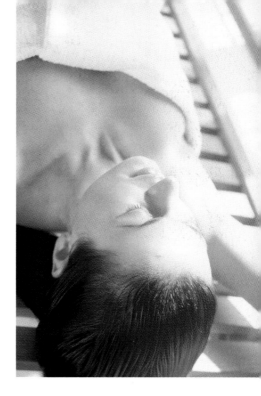

> Finally, you can try a specialist treatment at a beauty salon: algae baths, body wrapping, algonization (a combined treatment of algae wraps and electrical pulses).

KEY FACTS

* Algae retain the nutrients of the marine environment.

* Their most important property is their richness in iodine, which stimulates the thyroid gland.

* They stimulate the blood circulation and lymphatic system, working to reduce congestion in the areas affected by cellulite.

23

think about homeopathy

Homeopathy is not just about slimming but, as with similar areas of medicine, it can correct your metabolic trends and awaken dormant biological functions.

Everyone gains weight differently

Infinitesimal medicine is a new type of treatment that looks very closely at each patient, studying his or her tastes, aversions, pathological predispositions. A tendency towards weight gain is specific to each of us.

A homeopathic doctor is not only interested in your weight. He or she will also take into consideration the way in which you put on weight, changes in your appetite, your resistance to stress, your constitution and the parts of your body where you tend to gain weight etc.

Some examples

In homeopathy there are three types of constitution. Carbonics put on weight easily. Fluorines gain weight as they age. Phosphorics rarely put on weight despite having a healthy appetite. It is possible to correct the excesses that correspond to a constitution by prescribing the right remedy for each one. A homeopathic doctor might just as easily give you medicine to correct your hormonal functioning, help you to beat stress and improve kidney and liver functioning. This is good as a head start which, rather than replacing your diet, helps to make it more efficient.

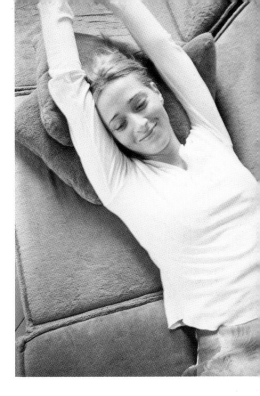

> This does not have anything to do with the subtle and highly individualized approach of homeopathy as practised today.

KEY FACTS

* Homeopathy looks into why each of us puts on weight

* Are you carbonic, fluorine or phosphoric? Your treatment depends on your constitution.

* Homeopathy can also improve the way your hormones function and aid elimination.

24

try appetite regulating granules

Some homeopathic remedies are particularly effective in helping dieters to reduce their appetite. Their effect is much more subtle than appetite suppressants.

Real hunger or compulsive urge

It's difficult to resist temptation when you're hungry. It's also difficult to hold out when you feel an urge that drives you to the refrigerator even when you're not hungry, because you're feeling depressed or affected by some strong emotion. We all have our weaknesses. Some can't resist chocolate, while for others its alcohol or salty foods. Each type has its own specific medicine.

● ● ● DID YOU KNOW?

> Some medicines also treat seasonal bulimic crises: if it's in winter that you most want to eat more, try Aurum or Sulfur; if it's in the Summer, try Gelsemium or Cina.

> In all events, take medicines at 9CH, 3 granules morning and evening. If you don't see any improvement after two weeks, consult a homeopathic doctor who will know how to refine the treatment.

Remedies that work

- You get so hungry at night that you have to get up to find something to eat: *Petroleum.*
- Hunger grips you in the night and you suffer from migraines: *Psorinum.*
- Your hunger drives you to eat very fast and this makes you feel good: *Anacardium orientalis.*
- You have irresistible urges to eat chocolate or drink alcohol: *Argentum nitricum.*
- You feel you want to eat when you're upset: *Ignatia.*
- You're a big eater and always feel hungry: *Antimonium crudum.*
- You always want a snack at around 11pm, before you go to bed: *Natrum carbonicum.*
- You get hunger pangs around 11am, towards the end of the morning, and get the urge to eat sugar: *Sulphur.*
- You get real hunger pangs, but they calm down after a couple of mouthfuls: *Lycopodium.*

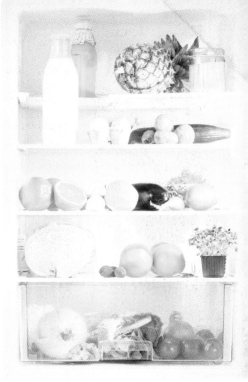

KEY FACTS

* Some homeopathic medicines can help to fight hunger pangs and cravings.

* They differ according to whether you get hungry at night or during the day, in winter or in the summer, if you prefer savoury or sweet foods.

25 use natural appetite suppressants

Some vegetable substances swell up in the stomach, creating a decoy for hunger. Plant and olfactory-based, appetite-suppressing chewing gums are available in some countries.

An indigestable gel: guar gum, extract of carob and some algae (i.e. carraghen and konakiu) have an interesting property – their fibres swell on contact with water and increase in volume almost instantly. Take two capsules with a large glass of water and you will feel as if you have a full stomach. These fibres cannot be broken down by the digestive juices and form a gel that eventually passes through the system. Efficient for big appetites but not good for compulsive eaters. You can also overcome some of the urge to eat by using ordinary chewing gum. Choose gums with non-absorbable sugars which help prevent tooth decay.

Powerful smells: smells go directly via the nose to the reptilian brain governing our emotions and vegetative life. Smell is the only sense not decoded by the cortex. It is directly linked to our instincts. The body can be duped into sending the brain an aroma instead of food, the principle behind olfactory boxes that you sniff when you feel a hunger pang.

KEY FACTS

* Some algae, guar gum or carob extract swell up in the stomach and curb hunger.

* Olfactory duping tricks the brain into thinking it has had nourishment.

26 take food supplements

Micronutrients play a role in all metabolic reactions, including weight loss. If you are deficient in vitamins, minerals, amino acids, fatty acids or trace elements you will lose weight more slowly.

Vitamins and trace elements: Vitamin B6 is found in many plant and animal foods and is important in the metabolism of amino acids. Vitamin C is found in fresh food and vegetables and is easily lost in cooking. It is essential for the synthesis of collagen. Iodine is vital for the effective operation of the thyroid gland that regulates the whole metabolism.

Amino acids and fatty acids: several amino acids play an active role in weight loss: the L-tyrosine, L-phenylalanine, L-carnitine, L-dopa and L-arginine. There are also dietary supplements that are adapted to aid weight loss that contain amino acids.
The properties of evening primrose oil have been well proven. In fact, the body uses the fatty acids of this oil to manufacture prostaglandin to help the body to shed excess pounds.

KEY FACTS

* Certain essential minerals, vitamins, trace elements, amino acids and fatty acids favour weight loss.

* Complex food supplements can avoid fatigue and depression.

27 prioritize eliminating toxins

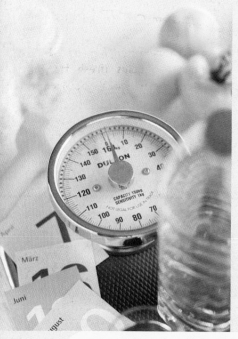

Before you start dreaming about losing weight, you need to help your body to rid itself of the toxins accumulated over the course of the previous months, or even years. You need to deep cleanse to ensure the success of your diet.

> Clay captures all the impurities that it meets on its way and allows you to eliminate them. Every evening, put a spoonful of powdered clay in a large glass of pure water, stir with a wooden spoon and leave to stand overnight.

● ● ● DID YOU KNOW?
> Help your body to rid itself of its toxins by following a clay treatment for three weeks.

Help the organs in their task

For you to lose weight, your body needs to burn its fat reserves. Unfortunately, toxins are also stored in these reserves with the result that at the same time as losing weight, your body releases a quantity of waste products that need to be eliminated. This won't be easy if it is already congested with toxins. Our cells are bathed in a liquid through which they receive nourishment and get rid of waste. This waste is evacuated in the organic liquids (blood and lymph). Various organs are involved in this process, to filter, recover and expel. A short, well-designed detox treatment will help them in their task. Your body, refreshed from the inside and renewed, will respond all the better to the weight-loss process.

Some treatment ideas

The vegetable detox: choose vegetables according to their specific depurative properties. Asparagus helps to drain the kidneys and the liver; peppers act as a general purifier; peas are full of cellulose so cleanse the digestive tract; French beans and spinach are mild laxatives. Eat mainly vegetables for one week, drink lots of water, stock or broth, infusions etc. Cut your intake of fat and protein to a minimum.

The liquid detox: for 24 hours (36 max), drink only liquids (fresh fruit juices, stock or broth, clear soups, soya milk, herbal teas).

KEY FACTS

Fat is a reservoir for the storage of toxins. When you lost weight, you free your body of these toxins.

Help your body to get rid of them, do a detox.

Choose between the vegetable detox, liquid detox or the clay detox.

> The following day, drink the clay-soaked water. If the taste doesn't put you off, stir before drinking to make your treatment even more efficient.

28

treat yourself to a slimming bath

Look after your figure while relaxing in the bathtub – just a dream, surely? No, it's true! Make the most of bath products containing plant extracts and speed up your diet while concocting luxurious baths that help the weight come off.

Relaxation, circulation, eliminating toxins

Even just a simple bath can be a relaxing experience. Beat the stress of the day and give your diet a boost. It's better to give yourself half an hour of perfumed relaxation than to raid the refrigerator. The heat of the water triggers vasodi-latation which activates the blood circu-lation and lymph system, particularly if you follow the bath with a quick cold shower on your legs, starting from your the feet and working upwards over the length of the calves and thighs. You will find that there will be a clear improvement in the elimination of toxins.

Plant extract slimming baths

Algae are widely used in ready-made preparations. But you can also prepare your own bath.

• **Anti-cellulite bath:** prepare a climbing ivy concoction. This plant contains phytoestrogens and saponosides that penetrate the tissue with a diuretic and depurative effect. It reduces inflammation of areas of cellulite and helps to reduce the thickness and has a beneficial impact on the blood circulation. Add 2 handfuls of fresh leaves to 2 litres (3$^1/_2$ pints) of cold water, boil for 5 minutes then leave to stand for 10 minutes. Strain, then add to your bath water.

• **Firming bath:** prepare a mixture of equal parts of fennel, rosemary, cypress and lemon essential oils. Take around ten drops of this liquid and add this mixture to a tablespoon of milk or bubble bath before turning on the taps to make sure it disperses properly. This bath also has a purifying effect.

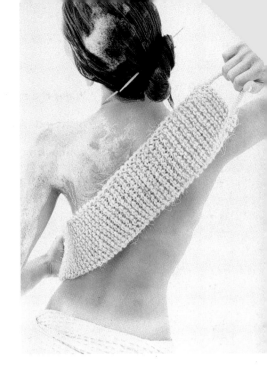

KEY FACTS

✳ Take a slimming bath instead of raiding the fridge.

✳ Don't have too hot a bath (38°C/100°F maximum) and don't stay in for any longer than 20 minutes at the most.

✳ Climbing ivy, rosemary, cypress, fennel and lemon essential oils are your slimming allies.

29

take exercise

If you want to lose weight it's not enough just to restrict your calorie intake, you also have to expend more energy. So, do some sport! Not only will you shed the pounds or kilos more easily, you will also reshape your figure.

Less fat, more muscle

The more you move, the higher your energy output. Even if sport doesn't directly make you lose weight, it is a vital part of any weight-reducing regime. After about 40 minutes your muscles need to renew their energy. They do this by drawing on fat reserves. Aside from this immediate result of fat burning there is also an increase in the muscular mass – so, less fat, more muscle – a more shapely, more elegant figure.

Less stress, fewer toxins, more oxygen

Playing sport regularly also helps to beat the stress that drives us to eat when we're not hungry in an attempt to calm our nerves, causing over-eating which then impacts on our metabolism by eventually slowing it down.

When you take exercise, you sweat: the body eliminates toxins. This is why you should always have a bottle of water to hand when exercising, to replace your water reserves.

So, after exercise the body is better oxygenated, the cells better nourished and the cardio-vascular system is strengthened. This whole series of benefits will increase the feeling of well-being and reduce the risks of compulsive bingeing.

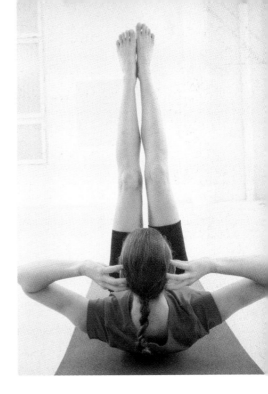

> This regular exercise is also important to improve the mental and emotional stability of people who are not feeling good about themselves: getting moving and feeling increasingly at ease with your body promotes self-acceptance. It's great for people who are shy or self-conscious.

KEY FACTS

* Sport is good for developing muscle mass.

* It also has other benefits: better oxygenation of the cells, reduction of stress.

* Exercise regularly and for extended periods so that the body can draw on its reserves.

30

choose the right sport for you

Not all sports are the same when it comes to weight loss. Choose an activity that gets your whole body moving and that involves long and regular energy expenditure and, above all, go for a sport that you enjoy.

Pleasure first

In order to be efficient, sport must be enjoyable. If you take up an activity that doesn't bring you any satisfaction, there's the risk that you'll give up. You should also choose a sport that fits into your lifestyle: take exercise somewhere that isn't too far away so that you don't run out of time. If you work irregular hours, opt for a sport that doesn't have to fit a specific timetable.

Moderate and regular effort

To help you to slim, sports must make your whole body work and use all your muscles. In this respect, swimming, speed walking, jogging and cycling are good. Roller skating is also excellent if you treat it as a sport. And why not try more original sports: rowing or cross-country skiing if you live in the mountains.

It is also important to choose an endurance sport as, to be efficient, the effort must be of average but sustained intensity. In short, in intense bouts of activity (i.e. weightlifting or sprinting) the muscles primarily burn sugars and only start to draw on fat reserves during sustained and regular exercise. You will feel the immediate benefit of a chain reaction: not only will you be burning fat but your body will use energy to finish the task at hand. Additionally, your increased volume of muscles will become 'greedier', so the overall expenditure will be higher.

> Also, many sports clubs require a medical certificate stating your fitness before you can register.

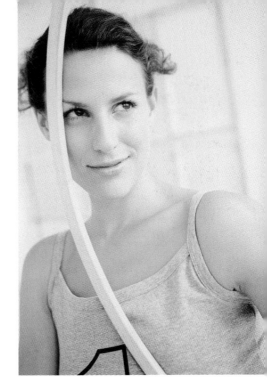

KEY FACTS

* Choose an endurance sport to burn fat.

* Play a sport that makes your whole body work: jogging, swimming, roller skating or rowing.

* Above all, opt for a sport that you enjoy and so won't give up on easily.

31

try lymphatic drainage

Lymphatic drainage is a must in the fight against cellulite. It's a pleasant and efficient technique as long as it is performed by a properly trained therapist. Elimination, firming up and slimming down are the order of the day.

About lymph

The circulatory system has three components: the arterial system, the venous system (both blood) and the lymphatic system. The latter helps the venous system eliminate waste from the metabolism. Running through this system is a thin, slightly gelatinous, whitish liquid called lymph. It contains urea, chlorine, glucose, lipids, proteins and organic acids. Lymph circulates through ducts equipped with little valves that work like locks to prevent liquid from flowing back into them. Part of the interstitial liquid in which our cells swim is drawn in to these ducts and is taken back to the top of the body where the bulk of the recycling system is located. On the way, it runs through lymph nodes that filter the liquid and recover some of the impurities for subsequent evacuation. What remains arrives at the level of the clavicles and joins the vena cava, mixing with the blood on its way to the lungs.

Deep, gentle movements

The one weak point of this otherwise well-oiled system is that it has no pump. In order to get back to the top of the body, lymph must fight gravity. Sometimes the system gets lazy, the lymph stagnates and waste accumulates. Cellulite starts to appear and the ankles and legs swell up. In the 1950s, Dr Vodder perfected a type of massage specifically designed to boost lymphatic circulation. It consists of a series of gentle but deep movements, (packs and pumps) that facilitate the opening of these 'lock gates' and improve lymph circulation. After a good lymphatic drainage treatment you generally need to pass water, which is a sign that the elimination process has speeded up.

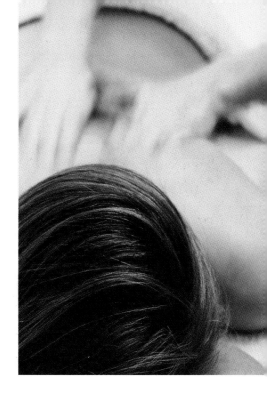

KEY FACTS

* Lymphatic drainage is a special massage that improves lymphatic circulation.

* It's very efficient in fighting cellulite and oedema.

* Lymphatic energy is a type of massage that centres on certain energy points.

32

Chinese medicine also covers weight loss. Some points situated on the energetic meridians can be used to boost metabolism, accelerating fat burning and waste elimination.

massage your feet and ankles

Fingertip massage

According to Chinese medicine, our body is stimulated by a vital energy that circulates through channels called meridians. By acting on specific points located along the course of these meridians, it is possible to improve the functioning of the body.

Acupuncture acts on these points with needles or moxas, little sticks with herbs at the end that are set alight. You can also stimulate them yourself by massaging them with your fingertips.

The points that aid slimming

Some points improve waste elimination and boost the overall metabolism of the body, increasing energy expenditure. Which is why it will help you to shed those extra pounds or kilos.

① The first point is located on the inside of your leg, about four fingers measure above the ankle and slightly towards the back.

② The second point is on the outside of your foot, about three fingers above your little toe.

③ The third one is on the bridge of your foot, about two fingers above your big toe.

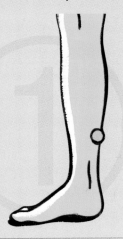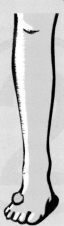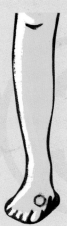

KEY FACTS

* Chinese medicine is also concerned with weight loss.

* Specific points accelerate elimination of toxins and boost the overall metabolism.

* You can stimulate these points yourself by pressing with your fingertips.

33 watch your hormone levels

Some forms of obesity are due to hormonal imbalances such as an under-active thyroid gland. Sex hormones are sometimes also the cause. Check with a specialist doctor to find out if this is true is your case.

The prime suspect – the thyroid gland: some people find it difficult to lose weight. In such cases, hormonal deficiency should be considered as a cause. The prime suspect is the thyroid gland which is responsible for numerous metabolic activities. When there is a shortage of thyroid hormones the body goes into economy drive, storing everything that it doesn't use. You feel tired, swollen, your hands and feet feel cold, and your hair becomes dull and lifeless.

Growth hormones, DHEA and progesterone… There are other hormones that play a role in weight gain, above all, sexual hormones in women. These are often temporary weight problems linked to menstruation and may be due to a lack of progesterone.

When it comes to hormone treatments however, you should never improvise. You need to consult a specialist doctor who will prescribe specific tests and advise treatment if deficiencies are identified.

KEY FACTS

* You may need to consider the possibility that you have an under-active thyroid.

* Only a specialist can check the status of your endocrine glands, particularly the thyroid gland.

34 try the Indian method

The ancient science of Indian health, Ayurveda, consists of purification treatments that enable you to cleanse your inner body and soul, to prepare for successful slimming. Exotic and efficient.

Healthy lifestyle, healthy body, lost pounds or kilos... Ayurveda is a traditional Indian medicine inspired by ancient precepts founded on a healthy lifestyle.
Ayurvedic treatments clean and purify the body as well as boosting the metabolism, which will all aid weight loss.

The typical treatment takes place at a specialist centre and lasts one week. The exclusively vegetarian diet borders on fasting. For the first few days the treatment concentrates on purifying the upper part of the digestive system (ingestions of warm salt water, massages). Then the lower part is purged with washes, always combined with massage. Finally, there are treatments with essential oils, steam baths, and relaxation and meditation sessions. You will leave feeling lighter than air.

● ● ● DID YOU KNOW?
> During treatments like this you will lose weight, but when you start eating normally again your body will re-constitute its reserves. Make sure you don't put it all back on by taking things slowly: reintroduce food groups one by one, carry on the diet one day per week (fruit and cooked vegetables) and take time to relax.

KEY FACTS

* Ayurvedic medicine has detox treatments that purify the body.

* These one-week treatments take place at a specialist centre.

* They combine cleansing treatments with massage, diet, relaxation and mediation.

35

spend some time by the sea

All thalassotherapy centres offer special slimming treatments. Don't expect miracles but they can effectively kick-start a diet. One week to acquire good habits – don't wait any longer – dive head first into slimness!

Great mineral wealth

The spas (Vittel, Evian etc.) were among the first to take up a position on the slimming market. Next came thalassotherapy centres. With a great wealth of trace elements and minerals, particularly in iodine, sea water is extremely good for this type of treatment which can boost the laziest metabolism.

These centres also offer diuretic treatments, as well as dietary training courses. Their customers can access alternative treatments such as shiatsu, sophrology and reiki among others.

Wet treatments and dry treatments

During the treatment, the minerals contained in the sea water penetrate the skin and help to reconstitute the body's reserves. Baths, whirlpools, jet showers and jacuzzis boost blood and lymphatic circulation and speed up the elimination of toxins. These are what we call 'wet treatments'. These are combined with 'dry treatments' such as massage, drainage and pressotherapy (a detoxifying treatment based on a compression system using inflating pumps to effect lymphatic drainage).

Don't forget sea mud and algae, which are particularly efficient when it comes to eliminating unwanted cellulite. They are principally used in the form of wraps. Of course, you aren't going to shed all your extra pounds on a one-week course. But it is a good way of changing your daily habits, modifying your diet, getting back into sport and learning to relax.

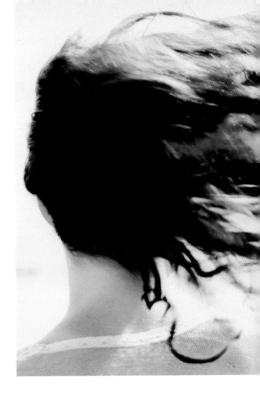

KEY FACTS

* Thalasso treatments are a good jump-start for a weight-loss programme.

* You can take advantage of both wet and dry treatments.

* These programmes are carefully carried out under medical supervision.

36

don't forget chromium

A recent discovery, the properties of chromium appear to be endless. It plays a vital role in metabolizing sugars, and therefore, in the accumulation of pounds or kilos.

Metabolizing sugars and fats

Chromium is one of the most recently discovered essential trace elements. Its role is vital for the proper functioning of the metabolism of fats and sugars, as well as for the regulation of blood cholesterol.

In order for the body to use the glucose available, it needs chromium. When present in sufficient quantity it participates in the regulation of sugar levels in the blood and economizes the production of insulin by the pancreas. The richer your diet in carbohydrates (sugar, sugary food, cereals, leguminous plants), the more important a high level of chromium. This is particularly important when you eat refined sugars as the chromium necessary for their assimilation is actually present in the base food (wholegrain cereals, sugar cane) but is lost in the refining process.

150 to 200 micrograms per day

Some of the signs of chromium deficiency are tiredness, high cholesterol and most of all, substantial weight gain. Nutritionists estimate that a good part of the population of the Western world have chromium deficiency. Their advice, in order to lose weight, is to take 150 to 200 micrograms of chromium a day.

There is no risk of overdose. You can also try to incorporate foods rich in chromium into your diet. Other than wholegrain cereals, eat brewer's yeast, liver, egg yolk and spices (thyme and black pepper). Organic (non-chemical) chromium is much better assimilated by the body.

> This sensitivity to industrial chromium is acquired when your hands come into contact with detergent products that reduce the natural protection of the epidermis.

KEY FACTS

* Chromium is vital for the metabolism of sugars and fats.

* When you have a chromium deficiency you feel tired and put on weight.

* Supplements of chromium are recommended because, in the West, deficiency is generalized.

37 drink floral remedies

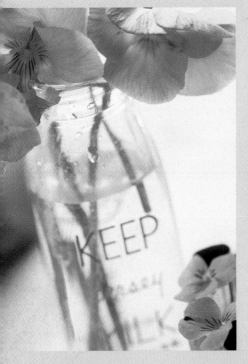

Floral elixirs perfected at the beginning of the twentieth century by Dr Bach can help you keep to your diet without anguish, fear or nerves... and without giving in to temptation!

> Every morning, use the pure elixi to prepare your dose for the day 2 drops in half a glass of pure water taken in small doses throughou the day.

Flowers balance our emotions

Dr Edward Bach dedicated his life to concentrating the whole essence of flowers and all their healing energy into these subtle extracts. This English doctor was convinced that all problems were rooted in emotional disorders. He established links between certain flowers and certain states of mind. A trained homeopath, he set out to naturally dilute the flowers, leaving the recently picked blossoms to rest in a small dish of pure water, exposed to the sun's rays. The result was the range of 38 Dr Bach floral elixirs.

Oak, walnut, cherry-plum or impatiens?

Try these elixirs to help you stick to your diet:

- **Impatiens:** calms people who eat quickly. They never feel full up and are never afraid to accept a second helping.

- **Cherry-plum:** is for people who are incapable of controlling their compulsive urge to eat.
- **Oak:** is for use by those who feel the need to eat to resist the onslaught of their surroundings.
- **Vervain:** suits people who go all the way, in so far as concerns their ideas, projects, books…and food.
- **Walnut:** helps to change habits and allows new eating behaviours to be introduced.

> You can also place 5 drops of elixir in your bath water. Treatment should last around 4 weeks.

KEY FACTS

* These gentle extracts of flowers harmonize our state of mind.

* They help to fight against the anxiety and nervousness that sometimes strike during a diet.

* Try oak, impatiens, vervain, cherry-plum and walnut.

38

opt for slimming – Eastern style

According to Chinese medicine, slimming depends on the way in which we transform food into energy. In order to stimulate this process, we must have faith in the needle.

A transformation problem

Each and every one of us gains our nourishment by simply absorbing foods. The process is a little more complicated in Chinese medicine, according to which we absorb four major types of food: solids, liquids and also the air and the emotions. These four, as a whole, nourish the cells as well as the vital energy that circulates in our bodies along the meridians. The primary meridian for weight problems is known as Chong Mo. It governs all the mutations of man, whether dietary or psychological. It is responsible for the digestion, since to digest a food is to transform it. If Chong Mo is functioning badly, the foods will not be correctly transformed into energy. This latter idea translates into something more tangible: extra pounds or kilos. Our resistance to transformation is also shown in our behaviour: we find it difficult to change, to adapt. To modify our diet, for example!

Needles and moxas

In order to re-establish the energetic balance of the body, acupuncture uses needles that are placed on specific points along certain meridians, either to stimulate the energy or to diffuse it. Acupuncture practitioners now use disposable, single-use needles to avoid any risk of contamination. They can also use moxas: sticks with herbs at the end that are lit like a cigar. The burning end is then brought as close as possible to a point to warm it.

> Yang foods are meat, cheese, fruits and red vegetables. All, of course, should form part of a balanced diet, adapted to your energetic profile.

KEY FACTS

* Extra weight is the result of the poor functioning of Chong Mo, the meridian charged with the transformation processes.

* Acupuncturists stimulate it with needles or moxas.

* Balance your meals according to the energy type of the foods.

39

do the bear!

If you want to balance your energies, you need to have faith in Qi Gong. These energetic exercises are the result of thousands of years of Chinese wisdom. Do the bear: you will feel better about yourself and help your body to lose weight.

Stimulate the meridian of the spleen

Problems of excess weight are sometimes linked in Chinese wisdom to poor circulation of energy in the meridian of the spleen. Try practising the bear position for ten minutes morning and evening in order to stimulate it.

A big, greedy animal

The bear is an animal symbolically linked to the Earth element, just like the meridian of the spleen, that governs the element. It likes sugar and honey but it has its feet firmly on the ground. Practising this position improves the circulation of energy in the meridian of the spleen and gives you more self assurance and confidence.

① Stand up straight with your feet together, arms flat against your sides.
② Bend your knees then stretch out your left leg to about twice the length of your shoulders.

③ At the same time, lift your arms up to waist level and your hands up to shoulder height, palms facing outwards.
• Bend your knees deeper so that your thighs are almost parallel with the floor.
• Push your hands forwards.

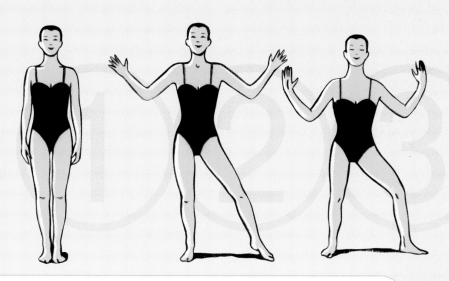

> During this exercise, you should first of all try to empty your mind of thoughts. Then concentrate on the centre of the palms of your hands and on the soles of your feet. Really become a fierce bear and throw an aggressive look ahead.

KEY FACTS

∗ Qi Gong energetic exercises help to stimulate the circulation of vital energy in the meridians.

∗ To lose weight, you need to stimulate the meridian of the spleen and take up the bear position.

40 try foot reflexology

A foot massage not only feels good, it can also serve a purpose. According to the principles of foot reflexology, you can massage specific points that correspond to the organs you wish to stimulate.

A map of the body on the sole of your foot: foot reflexology is based on the belief that we have reflex points on the soles of our feet that are linked to all the organs of the body. By massaging the soles of the feet, it is possible to stimulate and harmonize all the vital functions. Particularly, it is possible to boost the action of the thyroid gland by massaging the points that correspond to the neck area, the pituitary gland, the suprarenal glands and the genital organs.

The perfect massage: start by massaging the foot as a whole, moving up and down, working on the toes by kneading them one by one. Then, move on to the sole of the foot. Don't hold back from pressing down harder on tender points.

KEY FACTS

* Foot reflexology is a massage designed to boost the activity of the body.

* In order to lose weight, focus on the zones corresponding to the neck, pituitary gland, suprarenal glands and the genital organs.

case study

'I went on my first weight-loss diet when I was just 13. Work it out: that's 30 years now that I have been fighting my weight. I've learned to live with it! The moment I let my guard down, back come the pounds or kilos. That's just the way it is. But I have also learned that the struggle can be enjoyable and it is possible to make it less and less stressful. Of course, I had to learn to change my diet. I've got a really sweet tooth, so what I do is negotiate with myself on a tit-for-tat basis. Above all, I help my body to eliminate waste by any means possible. I play sport (not that much!) and I do a mono-diet in the spring and autumn, and I drink infusions made from plants with draining properties now and then. The most 'slimming' and enjoyable aspect is the massage: lymphatic drainage, energetic massage, I love all of that. I can't do without it. At home, I ask my husband to give me a massage every evening with essential oils. Once I even went on a thalassotherapy course with a friend. It was fabulous!'

41 »

» Learning to eat a healthy, balanced diet is vital. **Helping the body to eliminate waste is also very important.** But all of this won't be enough if your head refuses to let go of those extra pounds or kilos that have taken on an underlying meaning over the course of years.

»»» Changing your appearance is never easy, and a part of us sometimes resists this change. For your diet to be successful, **you also need to make peace with your image,** with your emotions and with your hidden desires.

»»»»» **This is often the start of a process of coming to terms with who you are** that goes much further than a few lost pounds or kilos!

60
TIPS

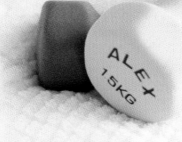

41

set yourself reasonable goals

Ah! Slimming… now there's a good opportunity for self-delusion and imagining yourself completely differently from the way you really are. And the less realistic you are, the lower your chances of success. It's better to look at the situation from a more reasonable angle.

Changing your body: a fantasy!

Losing a few pounds or kilos is not going to completely transform the way you look. If you have a big build and large bones, they will still be there afterwards. If you have short legs and a large chest, that's not going to change. What often happens is that in the desire to lose weight there is often a hidden desire to change your body shape completely. It's very important to get rid of this idea as,

● ● ● DID YOU KNOW?

> Top models generally have a BMI well below the norm. They are thin in the medical sense of the term. Some have a BMI score of below 15! Remember that if your weight is that low, your periods may switch off and you will be at greater risk of osteoporosis in later life.

> Don't try to look like them. Their extremely thin bodies are ideal for wearing any garment and can look good in any light and from any camera angle. This thinness is only attractive on a professional level.

if you don't, you're sure to fail. You will perhaps lose some weight, but the result will not measure up to your expectations and you will put it back on quickly.

Clarity and objectivity

It's better to get rid of your illusions and set yourself reasonable goals. First of all, in terms of weight: calculate your body mass index. All you do is to divide your weight in kilos by your height in metres squared. If, for example, you measure 1.60 m and weigh 54 kilos, it would be:

$$\frac{54}{(1.6 \times 1.6)} = 21$$

giving a body mass index (BMI) of 21 There are various websites that will do this calculation for you. A BMI above 18.5 is defined as thin, above 25, overweight. A score of above 30 denotes obesity. Consult your doctor who will know how to help you to find the causes of your weight gain and recommend appropriate treatment. If your score is between 25 and 30, you can attack the problem without assistance. Always avoid setting your goals too high. Take into account your age: it is normal to be a bit heavier at the age of 40 than you were at 20. Consider your build: logically, you will weigh more if you are big-boned. And don't feel that you need to lose those lovely curves that are part of your charm.

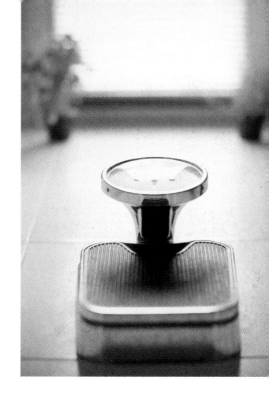

KEY FACTS

∗ The desire to lose weight sometimes masks a desire to change body shape. Remember, losing weight cannot change your height or build.

∗ You can get your body mass calculated by machine. A low electrical pulse is passed through the body giving accurate ratios of fat, water and muscle.

42

go back
to your
childhood

Every time you put food in your mouth
you are taking in, at the same time as
nourishment, memories, emotions, symbols,
fragments of your life – you need to think
about this to break free of your dependence.

Eating eases suffering

Newborn babies establish their first
relationship with the world through
food. Hunger causes them real physical
pain accompanied by anguish. Feeding
them is therefore a way of calming both
their physical and emotional suffering.
Not surprising then, that we sometimes
continue to hang on to these distant
feelings and that we seek comfort and
consolation in food, particularly warm

> Wine, for example, can remind you of your
grandfather lifting his glass at the end of a
family Sunday lunch, or perhaps, the blood of
Christ, the excesses of Bacchus, the warmth
of sharing, the promise of intoxication…

> All this on top of the numerous
minerals, antioxidants and vitamins it
contains. This is what we drink in
with each glass of wine we raise to
our lips. Stick to just one or two
though!

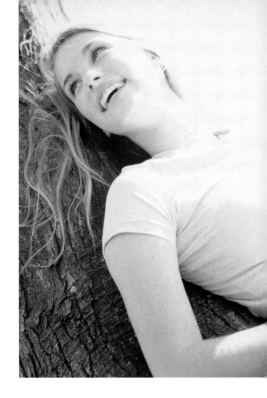

sugary food such as a newborn baby eats. All this is quite normal, but food is not the only source of emotional solace. If eating a chocolate bar calms your anxiety one day, but the next day you put on a Mozart symphony and the day after that you reach for a good detective novel, then you shouldn't worry.

Eating is a magic trick

If, on the other hand, you only seek comfort in food, it's time to ask yourself a few questions: Why? When did this emotional exclusivity form? What does food represent to you? What memories are linked to it? According to Dr Gérard Apfeldorfer, a psychiatrist specializing in eating behaviour, eating is a magic trick, 'A substance which is originally foreign to us comes through a complex process of alchemy to form part of us. It becomes us. Digestion is the act of transforming the non-self into the self. It's an intimate act!'
Every mouthful of food that we eat hides a world constituted by matter, of course, but also ancestral symbols, forgotten emotions and imperceptible echoes. It is these echoes that we need to update to get to the bottom of our dependence on food.

KEY FACTS

* Dependence on food goes back to our very first days of life.

* Food has a symbolic value that needs to be pinned down in order to get to the bottom of your eating behavioural problems.

43 learn to live with your image

If you want to lose weight, you must learn to look at yourself in the mirror. It's the best way of knowing where you're starting from, and measuring the path you travel every day towards the goal you have set yourself.

A chance glimpse of your reflection in a shop window: when you think you look fat, whether you are or not, you tend to avoid looking at your image. You look in the mirror less and less without even realizing it. And when by chance you catch a glimpse of your reflection in a shop window, you don't see yourself as you really are, or, at the very least, you see a distorted image of yourself.

Trust mirrors: you really have to learn to look at yourself. Give yourself some points of reference: first, look at yourself in the same mirror, in the same place, so that what you see is not distorted by external elements. Then, make an effort to put more mirrors around you – in the bathroom, in your bedroom etc. Try to look yourself in the face whenever you have the chance, in the hall before you go out, at a friend's house… there's nothing vain about it. It's just a way of reconciling yourself with your image.

KEY FACTS

* When you feel fat, you subconsciously get into the habit of avoiding looking at yourself.

* Put mirrors up around you, look at yourself when you're at a friend's house etc.

44 don't confuse weight loss with success

'When I'm thin, everything will be better...' When we harbour hopes such as these, we are paving the way for failure. Losing weight can bring you great satisfaction but it can't solve all your problems.

Pounds or kilos mask faults: 'When I'm slim, I'll have the courage to ask for a pay rise, I'll find the right man, I won't be shy any more...' A few excess pounds sometimes serve to cover up what we think are our faults or incompetence. We wait for our problems to melt away with the pounds or kilos.

Problems and extra padding: when you lose weight, old problems are updated. They re-emerge, stripped of any covering mask. You are thinner, of course, but that's all. And the fact of having lost weight is what makes us confront them. In a desire to avoid doing just this some people, subconsciously of course, prefer to put the weight back on. So try to measure clearly what you expect from your diet, without kidding yourself!

KEY FACTS

* You shouldn't ask more of a diet than it can realistically offer.

* Excess weight can sometimes act as a mask for problems.

45

analyze your attitude to food

Do you have a big or a small appetite? Are you a compulsive eater or a greedy gourmet? Do you have a sweet tooth or do you prefer savouries? Before you can adapt your diet to your tastes, you need to work out what type of eater you are.

Adapt your diet to your way of eating

Some people love to eat but know exactly when to stop. Others take no pleasure in eating unless everything is going smoothly. There are others, conversely, who can't stop eating when they are under stress. We all have our own eating patterns. If weight loss is to be maintained, it is important to learn to adapt these new eating habits to the

● ● ● D I D   Y O U   K N O W ?

> This logbook is important, above all, to verify your 'between-meal' eating habits. It's outside of set meal times that the majority of would-be slimmers tend to fall down.

> You have a snack, or a drink to pick you up or to relax, or you have a coffee with a little slice of cake or a piece of chocolate.

person that you are, with your own tastes and your own way of eating.

Write it down

The simplest way to confront your relationship with food is to keep a logbook. Take a notebook and divide each page into three columns. On the left, write down everything you eat, noting the time. In the right hand column, note down the most important events of the day. In the middle column, write down your state of mind in reaction to these circumstances: feelings of nervousness, joy, being upset etc. You will very quickly see the correlation between your activities, your emotions and your food urges. You will also see which are the foods that you eat most often. You may be in for a few surprises!

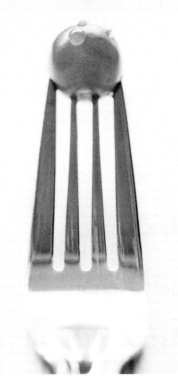

> And you hide the fact, only remembering what you ate for your previous meal.

KEY FACTS

* For sustainable weight loss, you must adapt these new eating habits to your way of eating.

* Discover your way of eating by keeping a logbook.

* If you do this, you will be able to see your 'between-meal' slip ups.

46

beat stress

Stress influences our eating habits and our metabolism. If you don't want to suffer the effects of stress, you must learn to protect yourself. Relaxation, plants and homeopathy are high on the agenda.

More appetite, more hormones

Stress influences weight gain by affecting our appetite. Some people eat more when they are under severe pressure, for reassurance. Learning to manage stress is an excellent exercise for regulating your appetite. But nervous tension also has a direct impact on the metabolism. When under stress, our body secretes a battery of hormones that prepare it for action. This tumult of hormones interferes with our basic metabolic functions.

The top stress-beaters

• **Relaxation:** (see Tip 47) can protect you from the effects of stress. There are other tools too:

• **Plants:** a valerian infusion can calm anxiety – place 1 tablespoon of roots in 250 ml (8 fl oz) of cold water, boil for 3 minutes and leave to infuse for 10 minutes. Official verbena will help you adapt to difficult situations – 50g per 1 litre (2oz per 1³/₄ pints) of cold water, soak for 10 minutes, boil for 10 seconds and leave to infuse for 10 minutes.

• **Homeopathy** can also be very effective in fighting stress.

> Most of the time we can't react physically by running away as fast as our legs will carry us, or by a fistfight. As a result, that barrage of hormones serves no purpose and causes problems along the way.

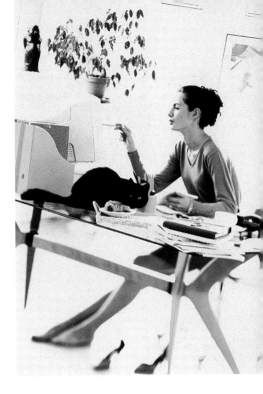

KEY FACTS

* Stress influences our appetite and our metabolism.

Beat stress by relaxing and having faith in plants and homeopathy.

* Our resources for dealing with stress are no longer adapted to modern life.

48

You can lose weight deliberately with greater speed when you are happy, relaxed and calm than in periods of grief or pain. So, learn to say yes to pleasure and happiness in your everyday life.

say yes to happiness

End poisonous friendships

Some people are good for us, while others can be aggressive, put us down and undermine our sense of worth. Sometimes we allow ourselves to be led into 'poisonous' relationships. Relational stress ensues, which is as disruptive as professional or family stress.

The psychological mechanisms that lead us to act in this way are complex.

Sometimes we surround ourselves with people who make us unhappy just because deep down we don't think we are worth any more than that. By means of compensation, to pacify, calm and sometimes to punish ourselves, we raid the cupboard or the fridge because food never lets us down. It doesn't measure the pleasure it gives us, it doesn't try to manipulate us… except when we step on the scales.

Cultivate self-esteem

The desire to slim is, more often than not, driven by one persistent feeling: we are not as we would like to be. We don't like ourselves and so we think that others don't like us either. The more failed slimming experiences we have under our belt, the more guilt erodes our feelings of self-esteem.

The way to break that spiral is to try to rebuild your self-esteem. Try to pinpoint your qualities and defects. Ask people you are close to and trust for advice. If you feel the need, seek the help of a therapist.

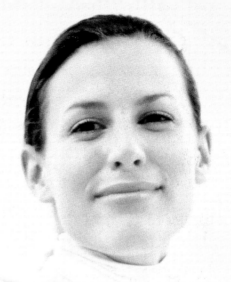

> If we perceive ourselves as 'unsatisfactory', we subconsciously do all we can to continue to conform to that deep-set image. And that includes putting weight back on that we have successfully lost!

KEY FACTS

* It is easier to lose weight when you are happy.

* Sometimes we don't allow ourselves to be happy: we tend to accumulate poisonous relationships.

* Recover your self-esteem by taking a good look at yourself.

49

manage your emotions

Emotional excesses are the Number 1 enemies of diets. A fit of anger, one big upset or anxiety attack, and we crack. Avoid the risk by learning to manage your emotions.

Our good resolutions are left by the wayside

Fear, anger, sadness, joy, surprise and disgust: six fundamental emotions o human beings that are shared by every one on the planet. These emotions are the worst enemies of diets. This i: because sometimes when we are con fronted by one of them, we go to pieces We are submerged in a cloud, a groun swell that makes us forget our objectives and our good resolutions – and that includes our slimming goals. We are not all equal when it comes to these extreme emotions. Some people suffer them only rarely whereas for others they are common occurrences. Everyone has their own strengths and weaknesses. One person may be incapable of resisting anger but will more easily control fear, while another will be thrown by unexpected turns of events and taken aback by sudden pleasures.

Identify, recognize and avoid

Avoid being overcome by your own emotions by learning to manage them. There are many techniques that allow this. They generally revolve around a central axis: first of all we must identify the emotions that disturb us, know how to recognize them when they happen

and implement strategies to enable us to avoid them. Sometimes, when the problem is very deep-rooted and is linked to an old emotional wound, our hidden memories must be explored to exhume the past causes of current emotional problems.

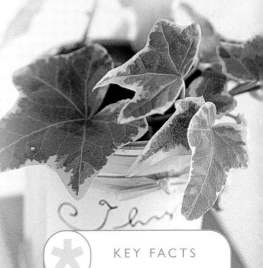

> Often just two or three minutes will be enough to find sufficient peace and to allow the worst storm to pass.

KEY FACTS

∗ Avoid being overcome by learning how to recognize that disturbing emotion, identify it and avoid it.

∗ Sometimes you need to look into the past to find the causes of current emotional problems.

50

imagine yourself fit and in shape

What if you were to replace your negative thoughts with positive thoughts? What if you were to concentrate on your successes instead of your failures? Positive thought sometimes has surprising results.

Allow your thoughts to wander

The principle of positive thought is simple. When we are relaxed, our minds are more receptive to images presented to them. All you need to do to make the most of this state, mid-way between dreaming and waking, is to allow your thoughts to wander, formulate some positive phrases, imagine yourself in ideal settings. It's a pleasant technique and more efficient than you think.

Psycho-corporal techniques also draw on the principles of positive thinking: sophrology, visualisation, the Silva method – each of these incorporates it into a broader mechanism. You can also practise positive thought at home, in the evenings, in bed before you go to sleep.

A typical session

Lie down in a dark, calm room and close your eyes. Make sure you won't be disturbed. Breathe deeply until you feel perfectly calm. Then repeat in your head a phrase that you have prepared in advance. For example: 'I can easily lose two pounds or one kilo a week, I feel light and in form, every week I get closer to my ideal weight.'
You can also imagine yourself as you dream of being at the end of your diet: you are with friends, you are wearing something that shows off your new shape, everyone is congratulating you, looking at you enviously.
It may seem like nothing but, little by little, the positive images and message will penetrate your mind, which will end up believing it. It will help you to attain your goals instead of putting spokes in the wheels.

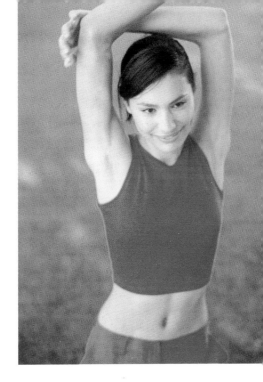

KEY FACTS

∗ Positive thinking rests on a simple principle: replace the negative messages that we constantly send out with more positive ones.

∗ You can also practise positive thinking in the evenings, in bed. If you do it regularly your mind will end up believing it!

51

dare to try NLP

Neuro Linguistic Programming (NLP) started in the 1970s in the USA. An extremely practical method, it aims to find the tools of your own success within you – whatever the nature of the problem, including weight problems.

A breakdown in communications... with yourself!

Neuro Linguistic Programming is a technique for communication with others and with yourself. Often, weight problems originate in misunderstandings between you and yourself. You lose sight of your real desires, you lack clarity as to your true motivations and as a result your goal remains out of reach. NLP is said to be very effective. It doesn't delve into your past or search for the hidden causes of current problems. It simply aims to help those who practise it to find in themselves the instruments of their own success, whatever the nature or degree of the problem, even something as 'trivial' as a weight problem.

The tools of NLP

We all have behaviours but these behaviours are not us. NLP puts forward some techniques to help us to free ourselves of these behaviours and to take up new attitudes more in line with our real desires: corporal and linguistic synchronization, dissociation, anchoring, location of strategies, identification of criteria. Some rather off-putting names for a series of complex techniques that must be practised under the guidance of a properly trained teacher.

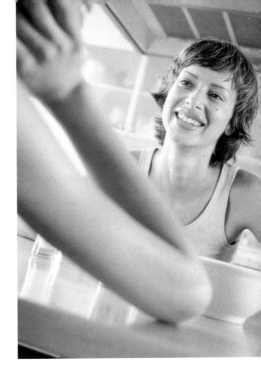

> The object is not to replace one problem with another: for example, becoming thin and depressed, thin and aggressive or thin and exhausted!

KEY FACTS

* NLP is a pragmatic technique that does not seek the cause of your problems in your past.

* It aims to identify our inappropriate behaviours and transform them.

* NLP should only be practised under the guidance of a properly trained teacher.

54

wage war on your hang-ups

Too thin, too fat, too much here and not enough there – we find it hard to love ourselves as we are. Hang-ups and complexes blight our lives and stop us from setting out calmly on an efficient weight-loss programme.

Parental models

There are some mornings when nothing seems to look good: you think you look dreadful in everything you wear, you don't like anything about yourself, you feel worthless, stupid, uninteresting. Stop! You really are suffering from a serious complex. You need to act fast to turn your ship around. Hang-ups and complexes are pointless and they ruin our lives. They are rooted in a distorted image we may have of ourselves that we inherited from our childhood, as none of us are actually born with any hang-ups. If parents are not wholly to blame, some of their attitudes may have encouraged the hang-ups. They may have dismissed our problems as trivial, over-protected us, undermined us in public or praised us so highly that we could never imagine living up to their expectations. Whatever the reason, the end results are the same.

A way out of your complexes

Excess weight is an ideal point of fixation for developing a complex: you can take action to get rid of the weight, so you feel really guilty about your inability to solve the problem. It's a frightening, efficient, vicious circle that sometimes prevents us from losing weight because if we were to lose the weight, we would lose the focus of our fixation. Suddenly we pile the lost pounds or kilos back on to recover our previous balance.

Before you begin to dream of losing weight, you must try to assess the true magnitude of your problem and evaluate the part your complexes play in that problem. If they constitute a considerable part of the problem, you should target your complexes before you target the excess weight!

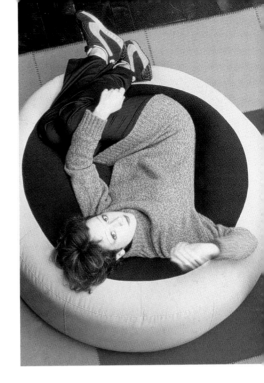

KEY FACTS

* Complexes are pointless and can blight our lives.

* Extra pounds or kilos are an ideal fixation point for our complexes. This is why we often regain the weight we have lost in order not to lose our mental balance.

55

When you have been overweight for a long time and it seems like nothing will shift those extra pounds or kilos, it's often because they serve a purpose in our mental balance. Now's the time to pay a visit to a specialized therapist.

put your faith
in a therapist

The underlying meaning
of surplus pounds and kilos

Those extra pounds or kilos can have an underlying meaning. Sometimes they appear in times of emotional shock or intense feelings, as if to protect us from the outside world. They can also serve as a shell into which we can withdraw from the world. Even if consciously we don't want to, our subconscious pushes us to

● ● ● DID YOU KNOW?

> Statistics have shown that cognitive-behavioural therapies give the best results in eating disorders.

> They can be a cure, particularly for actual bulimic behaviour.

cocoon ourselves in fat for its own reasons. Perhaps now is the right time to attack the underlying cause. Put your faith in a therapist.

Specialized therapists

There are therapists who are specialists in treating behavioural eating disorders. Psychiatrists and psychotherapists are the best armed to support you in your desire to lose weight. The longer you have been overweight, the more your mind will have organized itself around that fact. Perhaps your weight has secondary effects that you would never even have suspected. You can either choose a traditional therapist or a behavioural therapist. The former will endeavour to help you by looking into the hidden reasons behind your weight to make them fade, whereas the second will aim to modify your eating habits.

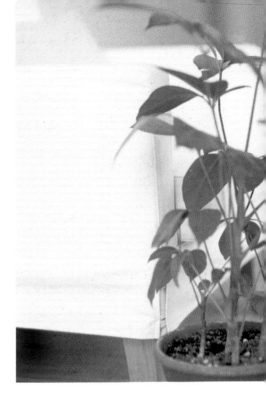

> **Work focuses both on the re-education of eating habits and the reconstruction of the self-image.**

KEY FACTS

* Our excess weight can have an underlying meaning

* Consulting a therapist can help with weight loss.

* Statistics show that cognitive-behavioural therapies give the best results with eating disorders.

useful addresses

» Acupuncture

British Acupuncture Council
63 Jeddo Road
London W12 9HQ
tel: 020 8735 0400
www.acupuncture.org.uk

British Medical Acupuncture Society
12 Marbury House
Higher Whitley, Warrington
Cheshire WA4 4QW.
tel: 01925 730727

Australian Acupuncture and Chinese Medicine Association
PO Box 5142
West End, Queensland 4101
Australia
www.acupuncture.org.au

» Homeopathy

British Homeopathic Association
Hahnemann House
29 Park Street West
Luton LU1 3BE
tel: 0870 444 3950

The Society of Homeopaths
4a Artizan Road
Northampton NN1 4HU
tel: 01604 621400

Australian Homeopathic Association
PO Box 430, Hastings
Victoria 3915, Australia
www.homeopathyoz.org

» Herbal medicine

British Herbal Medicine Association
Sun House, Church Street
Stroud, Gloucester GL5 1JL
tel: 01453 751389

National Institute of Medical Herbalists
56 Longbrook Street
Exeter, Devon EX4 6AH
tel: 01392 426022

» Massage

British Massage Therapy Council
www.bmtc.co.uk

Association of British Massage Therapists
42 Catharine Street
Cambridge CB1 3AW
tel: 01223 240 815

European Institute of Massage
42 Moreton Street
London SW1V 2PB
tel: 020 7931 9862

» Qi Gong

Qi Gong Association of America
PO Box 252
Lakeland, MN, USA
email: info@nqa.org

World Natural Medicine Foundation
College of Medical Qi Gong
9904 106 Street,
Edmonton AB T5K 1C4
Canada

» Relaxation therapy

British Autogenic Society
The Royal London
Homoeopathic Hospital
Greenwell Street
London W1W 5BP

British Complementary Medicine Association
PO Box 5122
Bournemouth BH8 0WG
tel: 0845 345 5977

'74 – 44 years

Editorial directors: Caroline Rolland and Delphine Kopff

Editorial assistant: Marine Barbier

Art editor: Guylaine Moi

Layout: G&C MOI

Final checking: Marie-Claire Seewald

Illustrations: Alexandra Bentz and Guylaine Moi

Production: Felicity O'Connor

Translation: JMS Books LLP

© Hachette Livre (Hachette Pratique) 2002
This edition published in 2004 by Hachette Illustrated UK, Octopus Publishing Group
Ltd., 2–4 Heron Quays, London E14 4JP

English translation by JMS Books LLP (email: moseleystrachan@blueyonder.co.uk)
Translation © Octopus Publishing Group Ltd.

A CIP catalogue for this book is available from the British Library

ISBN: 1 84430 077 3

Printed in Singapore by Tien Wah Press